Endoscopic Ear and Eustachian Tube Surgery

Editors

MUAAZ TARABICHI
JOÃO FLÁVIO NOGUEIRA

OTOLARYNGOLOGIC CLINICS OF NORTH AMERICA

www.oto.theclinics.com

October 2016 • Volume 49 • Number 5

ELSEVIER

1600 John F. Kennedy Boulevard • Suite 1800 • Philadelphia, Pennsylvania, 19103-2899

http://www.oto.theclinics.com

OTOLARYNGOLOGIC CLINICS OF NORTH AMERICA Volume 49, Number 5
October 2016 ISSN 0030-6665, ISBN-13: 978-0-323-46323-2

Editor: Jessica McCool
Developmental Editor: Alison Swety

Otolaryngologic Clinics of North America (ISSN 0030-6665) is published bimonthly by Elsevier, Inc., 360 Park Avenue South, New York, NY 10010-1710. Months of issue are February, April, June, August, October, and December. Business and Editorial Offices: 1600 John F. Kennedy Blvd., Suite 1800, Philadelphia, PA 19103-2899. Customer Service Office: 6277 Sea Harbor Drive, Orlando, FL 32887-4800. Periodicals postage paid at New York, NY and additional mailing offices. Subscription prices are $370.00 per year (US individuals), $765.00 per year (US institutions), $100.00 per year (US student/resident), $485.00 per year (Canadian individuals), $969.00 per year (Canadian institutions), $540.00 per year (international individuals), $969.00 per year (international institutions), $270.00 per year (international & Canadian student/resident). Foreign air speed delivery is included in all *Clinics'* subscription prices. All prices are subject to change without notice. **POSTMASTER:** Send address changes to *Otolaryngologic Clinics of North America*, Elsevier Health Sciences Division, Subscription Customer Service, 3251 Riverport Lane, Maryland Heights, MO 63043. **Telephone: 1-800-654-2452 (U.S. and Canada); 314-447-8871 (outside U.S. and Canada). Fax: 314-447-8029. E-mail: journalscustomerservice-usa@elsevier.com (for print support); journalsonlinesupport-usa@elsevier.com (for online support).**

Reprints. For copies of 100 or more of articles in this publication, please contact the Commercial Reprints Department, Elsevier Inc., 360 Park Avenue South, New York, NY 10010-1710. Tel.: 212-633-3874; Fax: 212-633-3820; E-mail: reprints@elsevier.com.

Otolaryngologic Clinics of North America is also published in Spanish by McGraw-Hill Interamericana Editores S.A., P.O. Box 5-237, 06500 Mexico D.F., Mexico.

Otolaryngologic Clinics of North America is covered in *MEDLINE/PubMed (Index Medicus), Current Contents/Clinical Medicine, Excerpta Medica, DIOSIS, Science Citation Index,* and *ISI/BIOMED.*

PROGRAM OBJECTIVE
The goal of the *Otolaryngologic Clinics of North America* is to provide information on the latest trends in patient management, the newest advances; and provide a sound basis for choosing treatment options in the field of otolaryngology.

LEARNING OBJECTIVES
Upon completion of this activity, participants will be able to:
1. Review the anatomy and function of the Eustachian tube.
2. Discuss preoperative and postoperative considerations, including outcomes, of endoscopic ear surgery.
3. Recognize methods in endoscopic management of conditions such as middle ear lesions, facial nerve surgery, and tympanoplasty, among others.

ACCREDITATION
The Elsevier Office of Continuing Medical Education (EOCME) is accredited by the Accreditation Council for Continuing Medical Education (ACCME) to provide continuing medical education for physicians.

The EOCME designates this enduring material for a maximum of 15 *AMA PRA Category 1 Credit*(s)™. Physicians should claim only the credit commensurate with the extent of their participation in the activity.

All other health care professionals requesting continuing education credit for this enduring material will be issued a certificate of participation.

DISCLOSURE OF CONFLICTS OF INTEREST
The EOCME assesses conflict of interest with its instructors, faculty, planners, and other individuals who are in a position to control the content of CME activities. All relevant conflicts of interest that are identified are thoroughly vetted by EOCME for fair balance, scientific objectivity, and patient care recommendations. EOCME is committed to providing its learners with CME activities that promote improvements or quality in healthcare and not a specific proprietary business or a commercial interest.

The planning committee, staff, authors and editors listed below have identified no financial relationships or relationships to products or devices they or their spouse/life partner have with commercial interest related to the content of this CME activity:
Matteo Alicandri-Ciufelli, MD, FEBORL-HNS; Jesus Franco Anzola, MD; Bernard Ars, MD, PhD; Mohamed Badr-El-Dine, MD; Adrianne Brigido; Marco Carner, MD; Yew Song Cheng, BM BCh; Michael S. Cohen, MD; Joris Dirckx, PhD; Anjali Fortna; Jacob B. Hunter, MD; Nicholas Jufas, MBBS, MS, FRACS; Seiji Kakehata, MD; Mustafa Kapadia, MD; Ruwan Kiringoda, MD; Elliott D. Kozin, MD; Daniel J. Lee, MD, FACS; Rudolf Leuwer, MD; Timothy Lian, MD, MBA, FACS; Daniele Marchioni, MD; Barbara Masotto, MD; Jessica McCool; Premkumar Nandhakumar; João Flávio Nogueira, MD; Nirmal Patel, MBBS, MS, FRACS; Livio Presutti, MD; Alessia Rubini, MD; Susan Showalter; Davide Soloperto, MD; Megan Suermann; Muaaz Tarabichi, MD; Domenico Villari, MD.

The planning committee, staff, authors and editors listed below have identified financial relationships or relationships to products or devices they or their spouse/life partner have with commercial interest related to the content of this CME activity:
Marc Dean, MD is a consultant/advisor for Acclarent, Inc. and BioInspire Technologies, and has stock ownership in BioInspire Technologies.
Brandon Isaacson, MD, FACS is a consultant/advisor for Stryker; KARL STORZ GmbH & Co. KG; Olympus Corporation of the Americas; Medtronic; and Advanced Bionics AG.
Dennis S. Poe, MD, PhD is a consultant/advisor for Accalarent, Inc. and OticPharma, Inc., with stock ownership in OticPharma, Inc.
Alejandro Rivas, MD is a consultant/advisor for Advanced Bionics AG; MED-EL; Cochlear Ltd.; Stryker; Grace Medical; Olympus Corporation of the Americas; and Acclarent, Inc.

UNAPPROVED/OFF-LABEL USE DISCLOSURE
The EOCME requires CME faculty to disclose to the participants:
1. When products or procedures being discussed are off-label, unlabelled, experimental, and/or investigational (not US Food and Drug Administration [FDA] approved); and
2. Any limitations on the information presented, such as data that are preliminary or that represent ongoing research, interim analyses, and/or unsupported opinions. Faculty may discuss information about pharmaceutical agents that is outside of FDA-approved labelling. This information is intended solely for CME

and is not intended to promote off-label use of these medications. If you have any questions, contact the medical affairs department of the manufacturer for the most recent prescribing information.

TO ENROLL
To enroll in the *Otolaryngologic Clinics of North America* Continuing Medical Education program, call customer service at 1-800-654-2452 or sign up online at http://www.theclinics.com/home/cme. The CME program is available to subscribers for an additional annual fee of USD 260.

METHOD OF PARTICIPATION
In order to claim credit, participants must complete the following:
1. Complete enrolment as indicated above.
2. Read the activity.
3. Complete the CME Test and Evaluation. Participants must achieve a score of 70% on the test. All CME Tests and Evaluations must be completed online.

CME INQUIRIES/SPECIAL NEEDS
For all CME inquiries or special needs, please contact elsevierCME@elsevier.com.

Contributors

EDITORS

MUAAZ TARABICHI, MD
Department of Otolaryngology; ENT Department, American Hospital Dubai, Dubai,
United Arab Emirates

JOÃO FLÁVIO NOGUEIRA, MD
Sinus and Oto Centro, Hospital Geral de Fortaleza, Fortaleza, Brazil

AUTHORS

MATTEO ALICANDRI-CIUFELLI, MD, FEBORL-HNS
Otolaryngology Department, University Hospital of Modena; Neurosurgery Department,
New Civil Hospital Sant'Agostino-Estense, Baggiovara, Modena, Italy

JESUS FRANCO ANZOLA, MD
Otolaryngology & Skull Base Surgery, Caracas Medical Center, Caracas, Distrito Federal
Venezuela

BERNARD ARS, MD, PhD
University of Namur, Faculty of Sciences, Namur, Belgium

MOHAMED BADR-EL-DINE, MD
Otolaryngology Department, University Hospital of Alexandria, Rouschdy, Alexandria,
Egypt

MARCO CARNER, MD
Otolaryngology Department, University Hospital of Verona, Verona, Italy

YEW SONG CHENG, BM BCh
Department of Otolaryngology, Massachusetts Eye and Ear Infirmary; Department of
Otology and Laryngology, Harvard Medical School, Boston, Massachusetts

MICHAEL S. COHEN, MD
Assistant Professor of Otolaryngology, Harvard Medical School; Director, Pediatric
Hearing Loss Clinic, Division of Pediatric Otolaryngology, Massachusetts Eye and Ear
Infirmary, Boston, Massachusetts

CHARLES R.J. DAULTREY, MRCS
University Hospital Birmingham, Birmingham, United Kingdom

MARC DEAN, MD
Clinical Assistant Professor, Department of Otolaryngology-Head and Neck Surgery,
Louisiana State University Health Sciences Center, Shreveport, Louisiana; Director,
Otorhinologic Research Institute, Fort Worth, Texas

JORIS DIRCKX, PhD
Laboratory of Biomedical Physics, University of Antwerp, Antwerp, Belgium

JACOB B. HUNTER, MD
Neurotology Fellow, Department of Otolaryngology-Head and Neck Surgery, Vanderbilt University Medical Center, Nashville, Tennessee

RICHARD M. IRVING, FRCS
University Hospital Birmingham, Birmingham, United Kingdom

BRANDON ISAACSON, MD, FACS
Associate Professor, Department of Otolaryngology–Head and Neck Surgery, University of Texas–Southwestern Medical Center, Dallas, Texas

NICHOLAS JUFAS, MBBS, MS, FRACS
Discipline of Surgery, Kolling Deafness Research Centre, Sydney Medical School, University of Sydney; Macquarie University; Sydney Endoscopic Ear Surgery (SEES) Research Group, Sydney, New South Wales, Australia

SEIJI KAKEHATA, MD
Otolaryngology Department, University Hospital of Yamagata, Yamagata, Japan

MUSTAFA KAPADIA, MD
Department of Otolaryngology, American Hospital Dubai, Dubai, United Arab Emirates

RUWAN KIRINGODA, MD
Clinical Fellow, Department of Otolaryngology, Massachusetts Eye and Ear Infirmary; Department of Otology and Laryngology, Harvard Medical School, Boston, Massachusetts

ELLIOTT D. KOZIN, MD
Resident, Department of Otolaryngology, Massachusetts Eye and Ear Infirmary; Department of Otology and Laryngology, Harvard Medical School, Boston, Massachusetts

DANIEL J. LEE, MD, FACS
Associate Professor, Department of Otolaryngology, Massachusetts Eye and Ear Infirmary; Department of Otology and Laryngology, Harvard Medical School, Boston, Massachusetts

RUDOLF LEUWER, MD
Professor of ORL, Head of ENT Department, Medical Director, HELIOS Hospital Krefeld, Lutherplatz, Krefeld, Germany

TIMOTHY LIAN, MD, MBA, FACS
Professor and Vice Chair of Clinical Affairs, Department of Otolaryngology-Head and Neck Surgery, Louisiana State University Health Sciences Center, Shreveport, Louisiana

DANIELE MARCHIONI, MD
Otolaryngology-Head and Neck Surgery Department, University Hospital of Verona, Verona, Italy

BARBARA MASOTTO, MD
Neurosurgery Department, University Hospital of Verona, Verona, Italy

JOÃO FLÁVIO NOGUEIRA, MD
Sinus and Oto Centro, Hospital Geral de Fortaleza, Fortaleza, Brazil

NIRMAL PATEL, MBBS, MS, FRACS
Discipline of Surgery, Kolling Deafness Research Centre, Sydney Medical School, University of Sydney; Macquarie University; Sydney Endoscopic Ear Surgery (SEES) Research Group, Sydney, New South Wales, Australia

DENNIS S. POE, MD, PhD
Professor of Otolaryngology, Harvard Medical School; Department of Otolaryngology and Communications Enhancement, Boston Children's Hospital, Boston, Massachusetts

LIVIO PRESUTTI, MD
Otolaryngology Department, University Hospital of Modena, Modena, Italy

JAMES W. RAINSBURY, FRCS
University Hospital Birmingham, Birmingham; Derriford Hospital, Plymouth, United Kingdom

ALEJANDRO RIVAS, MD
Associate Professor, Department of Otolaryngology-Head and Neck Surgery, Vanderbilt University Medical Center, Nashville, Tennessee

ALESSIA RUBINI, MD
Otolaryngology Department, University Hospital of Verona, Verona, Italy

DAVIDE SOLOPERTO, MD
Otolaryngology Department, University Hospital of Verona, Verona, Italy

MUAAZ TARABICHI, MD
Department of Otolaryngology; ENT Department, American Hospital Dubai, Dubai, United Arab Emirates

DOMENICO VILLARI, MD
Otolaryngology Department, University Hospital of Modena, Modena, Italy

Contents

> The eustachian tube consists of 2 compartments: the Rüdinger's safety canal
> and the auxiliary gap. It is surrounded by a cartilaginous wall on the craniome-
> dial side and a membranous wall on the inferolateral side. The eustachian
> tube cartilage is firmly attached to the skull base by the lateral and the medial
> suspensory ligaments, which are separated by the medial Ostmann fat pad.
> The function of the isometric tensor veli palatini muscle is modulated by hy-
> pomochlia, which have an influence on the muscular force vectors.

 Video content accompanies this article at http://www.oto.theclinics.
com.

> The protympanum, a final common pathway between the tympanic cavity
> and external environment, is gaining relevance due to the ease and
> completeness of visualization with angled endoscopes. Two primary confor-
> mations are described, quadrangular and triangular, and new anatomic
> structures such as the protiniculum, subtensor recess, and protympanic
> spine are defined. Surgical relevance of the protympanum is described
> with respect to ventilation, cholesteatoma, cerebrospinal fluid leak, otic neu-
> ralgia, and surgical access to the eustachian tube.

> The fibrocartilaginous eustachian tube is part of a system of contiguous
> organs including the nose, palate, rhinopharynx, and middle ear cleft.
> The middle ear cleft consists of the tympanic cavity, which includes the
> bony eustachian tube (protympanum) and the mastoid gas cells system.
> The tympanic cavity and mastoid gas cells are interconnected and allow
> gaseous exchange and pressure regulation. The fibrocartilaginous eusta-
> chian tube is a complex organ consisting of a dynamic conduit with its mu-
> cosa, cartilage, surrounding soft tissue, peritubal muscles (ie, tensor and
> levator veli palatine, salpingopharyngeus and tensor tympani), and supe-
> rior bony support (the sphenoid sulcus).

Paralleling the introduction of endoscopes for sinus surgery more than two decades ago, otology is facing a similar paradigm shift in the use of endoscopes to perform ear surgery. The wide-angle and high-resolution image provided by endoscopes allows for improved visualization of the tympanic cavity using minimally invasive surgical portals. Incorporating endoscopic ear surgery into otologic practice is challenging. A graduated and step-wise introduction of EES to otologic surgery is recommended to ensure safe and successful implementation.

 Video content accompanies this article at http://www.oto.theclinics.com.

The endoscope has transformed the way we observe, understand, and treat chronic ear disease. Improved view, exclusive transcanal techniques, assessment of ventilation routes, and mastoid tissue preservation have led to decreased morbidity and functional enhancement of minimally invasive reconstruction of the middle ear. The philosophical identity of endoscopic ear surgery is evolving; new research, long-term results, and widespread acknowledgement of its postulates will undoubtedly define its role in otology.

The main application of endoscopic surgery relies on the middle ear cholesteatoma surgical treatment, although for a definitive validation and acceptance by scientific community, long-term results are needed about recurrent and residual rates of the pathology. The aim of this article is to analyze the single institution experience with the long-term results of surgical treatment of attic cholesteatoma.

Endoscopic ear surgery (EES) provides several advantages compared with traditional binocular microscopy, including a wide-field view, improved resolution with high magnification, and visual access to hidden corridors of the middle ear. Although binocular microscopic-assisted surgical techniques remain the gold standard for most otologists, EES is slowly emerging as a viable alternative for performing otologic surgery at several centers in the United States and abroad. In this article, we evaluate the current body of literature regarding EES outcomes, summarize our EES outcomes at the Massachusetts Eye and Ear Infirmary, and compare these results with data for microscopic-assisted otologic surgery.

Special Article

This article discusses conservatively managed tumors, whether larger tumors at presentation are more likely to grow, and whether position at presentation corresponds with growth. A review is presented of more than
900 patients managed at Queen Elizabeth Hospital, Birmingham, between
1997 and 2012. Tumors were arbitrarily divided into 3 groups: intracanalicular (IC), and extracanalicular (EC) tumors measuring 1 to 10 mm or 11 to
20 mm at the cerebellopontine angle. This series shows that larger EC tumors grow faster than IC tumors and that EC tumors overall at presentation are more likely to grow than IC tumors.

OTOLARYNGOLOGIC CLINICS
OF NORTH AMERICA

THE CLINICS ARE AVAILABLE ONLINE!
Access your subscription at:
www.theclinics.com

Preface

Functional Endoscopic Chronic Ear Surgery: A New Horizon

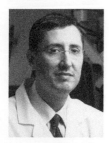 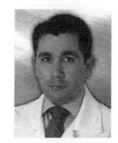

Muaaz Tarabichi, MD   João Flávio Nogueira, MD
Editors

Microscopic techniques, introduced to clinical practice in the late 1950s, have changed the character and outcomes in chronic ear surgery. We believe that the endoscope offers a similar "game-changing" impact on the management of our patients. No longer are we limited to fixing the battle scars of the chronic ear by closing perforations and reducing retraction. The improved access to the tympanic cavity and proximal Eustachian tube will allow us a better understanding of the primary disease process: impaired ventilation. The previous issue of *Otolaryngologic Clinics of North America* on endoscopic ear surgery aimed to introduce readers to the basics of this technique and was very well received. This follow-up issue focuses on re-establishing ventilation of the air cell system of the temporal bone, the most important predictor of restoring function to the ear.

Muaaz Tarabichi, MD
American Hospital Dubai
PO Box 5566
Oud Mehta Road
Dubai, United Arab Emirates

João Flávio Nogueira, MD
Sinus & Oto Centro
Hospital Geral de Fortaleza
Rua Dr. José Furtado, 1480
60822-300 Fortaleza, Brazil

E-mail addresses:
mtarabichi@ahdubai.com (M. Tarabichi)
joaoflavioce@hotmail.com (J.F. Nogueira)

Otolaryngol Clin N Am 49 (2016) xv
http://dx.doi.org/10.1016/j.otc.2016.07.012
0030-6665/16/© 2016 Published by Elsevier Inc.

Editorial

The Eustachian Tube Redefined

 CrossMark

It consists of two parts: the first solidly connected with the temporal bone, close to the tympanic cavity; the second soft, partly ligamentous, partly cartilaginous, directed towards the nasopharynx.
—*Bartholomeus Eustachius, Epistola de Auditus Organis (Examination of the Organ of Hearing), 1562, Rome*

Since its first description by Eustachius, the concept of the Eustachian tube as partly bony structure has taken deep roots in our understanding of its anatomy, function, and possible dysfunction. Microscopic and gross anatomical observations of the "bony tube" have made a distinction between "the protympanum," a tympanic cavity structure, and a more anterior and inaccessible "bony Eustachian tube." Endoscopic observation of that area allows a very different view of anatomy and renders this distinction arbitrary and irrelevant.

While the protympanum was once a difficult-to-access region of the middle ear, the adoption of middle-ear endoscopes and angled instrumentation has made direct viewing and access feasible. Indeed, by observing the protympanum from this perspective, it is clear that the bony Eustachian tube and the protympanum are essentially one and the same.

The Eustachian tube as viewed endoscopically does not have a bony portion. It is a fibrous/cartilaginous structure that stretches from the nasopharynx to the most anterior part of the tympanic cavity (the protympanum). Its two openings are strikingly similar cufflike protrusions into the relevant space. This new understanding allows a more clear and distinct anatomical description of an area that is increasingly accessible for surgical interventions.

Muaaz Tarabichi, MD
American Hospital Dubai
PO Box 5566
Oud Mehta Road
Dubai, United Arab Emirates

Dennis S. Poe, MD, PhD
Harvard Medical School
243 Charles Street
Boston, MA 02114, USA

Department of Otolaryngology
and Communications Enhancement
Boston Children's Hospital, BCH 3129
300 Longwood Avenue
Boston, MA 02115, USA

Otolaryngol Clin N Am 49 (2016) xvii–xx
http://dx.doi.org/10.1016/j.otc.2016.07.013
0030-6665/16/© 2016 Published by Elsevier Inc.

xviii   Editorial

João Flávio Nogueira, MD
Sinus and Oto Centro–Hospital Geral de Fortaleza
Rua Dr. José Furtado, 1480
60822-300 Fortaleza, Brazil

Matteo Alicandri-Ciufelli, MD, FEBORL-HNS
Otolaryngology Department
University Hospital of Modena
Via del Pozzo 71
41100 Modena, Italy

Neurosurgery Department
New Civil Hospital Sant'Agostino-Estense
Stradello Baggiovara 53
41126 Baggiovara (MO), Italy

Mohamed Badr-El-Dine, MD
Otolaryngology Department
University Hospital of Alexandria
36 Rouschdy Street #6
Rouschdy, Alexandria, Egypt

Michael S. Cohen, MD
Harvard Medical School
243 Charles Street
Boston, MA 02114, USA

Pediatric Hearing Loss Clinic
Division of Pediatric Otolaryngology
Massachusetts Eye and Ear Infirmary
Boston, MA, USA

Marc Dean, MD
Department of Otolaryngology–Head and Neck Surgery
Louisiana State University Health Sciences Center
Shreveport, LA, USA

Otorhinologic Research Institute
Fort Worth, TX, USA

Brandon Isaacson, MD, FACS
Department of Otolaryngology–Head and Neck Surgery
University of Texas–Southwestern Medical Center
5323 Harry Hines Boulevard
Dallas, TX 75390-9035, USA

Nicholas Jufas, MBBS, MS, FRACS
Kolling Deafness Research Centre
University of Sydney and
Macquarie University
Discipline of Surgery
Sydney Medical School
Sydney, Australia

Daniel J. Lee, MD, FACS
Department of Otolaryngology
Massachusetts Eye and Ear Infirmary
Boston, MA, USA

Department of Otology and Laryngology
Harvard Medical School
243 Charles Street
Boston, MA 02114, USA

Rudolf Leuwer, MD
ENT Department
HELIOS Hospital Krefeld
Lutherplatz 40
47805 Krefeld, Germany

Daniele Marchioni, MD
Otolaryngology Department
University Hospital of Verona
Verona, Italy

Nirmal Patel, MBBS, MS, FRACS
Kolling Deafness Research Centre
University of Sydney and
Macquarie University
Discipline of Surgery
Sydney Medical School
Sydney, Australia

Sydney Endoscopic Ear Surgery Research Group
Suite A12
24-32 Lexington Drive
Bella Vista, New South Wales 2153, Australia

Livio Presutti, MD
Otolaryngology Department
University Hospital of Modena
Via del Pozzo 71
41100 Modena, Italy

Alejandro Rivas, MD
Department of Otolaryngology–Head and Neck Surgery
Vanderbilt University Medical Center
1215 21st Avenue South, Suite 7209
Nashville, TN 37232, USA

E-mail addresses:
mtarabichi@ahdubai.com (M. Tarabichi)
Dennis.Poe@childrens.harvard.edu (D.S. Poe)
joaoflavioce@hotmail.com (J.F. Nogueira)
matteo.alicandri@hotmail.it (M. Alicandri-Ciufelli)
mbeldine@yahoo.com (M. Badr-El-Dine)
Michael_Cohen@meei.harvard.edu (M.S. Cohen)
marc.dean@gmail.com (M. Dean)

Brandon.isaacson@utsouthwestern.edu (B. Isaacson)
njufas@gmail.com (N. Jufas)
Daniel_Lee@meei.harvard.edu (D.J. Lee)
rudolf.leuwer@helios-kliniken.de (R. Leuwer)
marchionidaniele@yahoo.it (D. Marchioni)
nirmal.p.patel@gmail.com (N. Patel)
presutti.livio@policlinico.mo.it (L. Presutti)
alejandro.rivas@vanderbilt.edu (A. Rivas)

Anatomy of the Eustachian Tube

Rudolf Leuwer, MD

KEYWORDS

- Eustachian tube cartilage • Rüdinger safety canal • Auxiliary gap • Ostmann fat pad
- Tubal supensory ligaments • Tensor veli palatini muscle • Medial pterygoid muscle
- Salpingopharyngeal muscle

KEY POINTS

- The opening of the eustachian tube, provided by the contraction of the tensor veli palatini muscle, is limited to Rüdinger safety canal.
- The contraction of the tensor veli palatini muscle is almost completely isometric; it depends on hypomochlia, which modulate the muscular force vectors.
- Due to their fibromuscular interconnections on both sides of the Weber-Liel fascia, tensor veli palatini muscle and medial pterygoid muscle form a functional unit.

The eustachian tube consists of 2 different portions: an osseous posterolateral and a fibrocartilaginous anteromedial portion. The osseous portion is grossly formed by the petrous part of the temporal bone, the flexible fibrocartilaginous portion by the tubal cartilage, and its surrounding tissue. The active eustachian tube function is located in the fibrocartilaginous portion. This portion is connected to the skull base by suspensory ligaments.

SPATIAL ORIENTATION

The longitudinal axis of the tube forms an angle with the mediosagittal plane as well as with the horizontal plane.[1] The angle between the longitudinal axis of the cartilaginous part of the eustachian tube and the mediosagittal plane in adults is about 45° on average. In infants, it is only about 10°.[2] The average angle between the Frankfurt horizontal plane (orbitomeatal plane) and the tubal longitudinal axis in adults is about 35°.[1]

LENGTH

The total length of the eustachian tube ranges between 31 and 44 cm[3,4] in adults. Its length in newborns measures only about one-half of the adult's.[5] The length of the

---

Declaration of Conflicts: There are no commercial or financial conflicts of interest. There are no funding sources for the underlying scientific work.
ENT-department, HELIOS Hospital Krefeld, Lutherplatz 40, Krefeld 47805, Germany
E-mail address: rudolf.leuwer@helios-kliniken.de

Otolaryngol Clin N Am 49 (2016) 1097–1106
http://dx.doi.org/10.1016/j.otc.2016.05.002
0030-6665/16/$ – see front matter

osseous part is about one-third; the length of the fibrocartilaginous part is about two-thirds of its total length. There is no sharp borderline between the osseous and the fibrocartilaginous portion for the cartilage extends into the roof of the osseous part.[6] The tubal cartilage ends posterolaterally to the isthmus, which is the narrowest point in the tubal lumen. According to Zöllner,[4] the distance between the pharyngeal orifice and the isthmus measures 24 to 28 mm. Rüdinger[7] observed a fibrocartilaginous mass connecting the bone and the hyaline cartilage; this is the reason why there is a difference between the length of the cartilage, which is about 31.2 mm, and the fibrocartilaginous portion of the eustachian tube, which is about 26 mm. Pahnke even observed cartilage reaching the tympanic orifice of the tube.[1]

COMPARTMENTS

On a frontal 2-dimensional view, **Fig. 1** depicts the main structures contributing to the functional eustachian tube anatomy.

The fibrocartilaginous portion of the eustachian tube is almost completely surrounded by the tubal cartilage and by the tensor veli palatini muscle.[8] Both structures form the cartilaginous and the muscular wall of the eustachian tube.[7]

Cartilage

With respect to the eustachian tube function, the cartilage is a very important structure, because it forms the luminal frame of the tube.[8] Looking at the cross-section of the eustachian tube cartilage, its shape resembles a shepherd's crook,[9] consisting of a dome with a short lateral lamina and a long medial lamina. The lateral lamina has a mean height of 1.8 mm at its largest extension, and the medial lamina has a mean maximum height of 5.1 mm. This maximum height of both laminae can be found at about 6.6 mm behind the pharyngeal orifice. The size and shape of the lateral lamina are much more constant than that of the medial lamina. By means of MRI studies of the eustachian tube, Oshima and colleagues[8] could demonstrate a wide individual variety especially of the medial lamina. They concluded that this could have potential implications for eustachian tube surgery. Pahnke[10] also described this variety, which he found in an anatomic specimen. In about 25% of his specimen, the lower end of the medial lamina formed a hook around the lower portion of the eustachian tube lumen. The thickness of the medial and lateral lamina in the middle portion is approximately equal. In comparison to the medial lamina, the lateral lamina, however, becomes thinner toward both orifices.[10]

According to Bluestone,[9] the elasticity of the tubal cartilage is comparable to that of the pinna and the nasal cartilage. This elasticity, which is higher in adults than in infants,[11] is crucial for the reset forces after the contraction of tensor veli palatini muscle.

Lumen

Fig. 2 is a copy of an original illustration by Rüdinger.[7] It shows his cross-sectional view of the tubal lumen. Rüdinger distinguishes between 2 zones of the tubal lumen:

- A cranial half-cylindrical space, which today is called the "Rüdinger safety canal." This space is situated between the lateral and the medial lamina of the cartilage and is filled with mucus or air. Its diameter is about 0.5 mm, and it is found in about 85% of the adults. Most probably this space is always open.[10] The safety canal probably warrants pressure equalization and ventilation function of the eustachian tube.[12]
- Under the safety canal, there is a gap that is mainly surrounded by the muscular or membranous wall of the eustachian tube and partly by the medial lamina of the

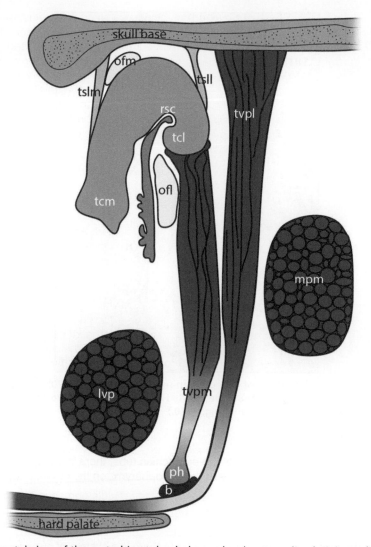

Fig. 1. Frontal view of the eustachian tube. b, bursa; lvp, levator veli palatini muscle; mpm, medial pterygoid muscle; ofl, lateral Ostmann fat pad; ofm, medial Ostmann fat pad; ph, pterygoid hamulus; rsc, Rüdinger's safety canal; tcl, tubal cartilage, lateral lamina; tcm, tubal cartilage, medial lamina; tsll, lateral tubal suspensory ligament; tslm, medial tubal suspensory ligament; tvpl, tensor veli palatini muscle, lateral layer; tvpm, tensor veli palatini muscle, medial layer.

cartilage. Rüdinger[7] called this gap the "auxiliary gap." The figure shows mucosal folds in the lower medial wall of the auxiliary gap. These inconstant folds were also described by Sando and colleagues[13] and by Ozturk and colleagues.[14] These so-called microturbinates seem to contribute to the mucociliary clearance and to the protection function of the eustachian tube.

The height of the lumen widely differs: in the petrous portion of the temporal bone, it is about 3.5 mm; 6 to 7 mm proximally to the pharyngeal orifice it is 6 to 10 mm.[1,9]

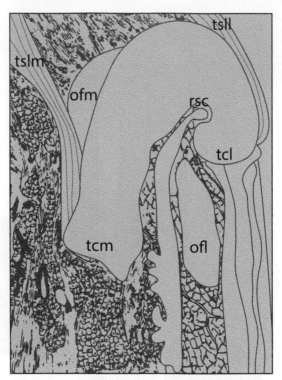

Fig. 2. Rüdinger's illustration of the human eustachian tube (1870). (*Adapted from* Rüdinger N. Vergleichende Anatomie und Histologie der Ohrtrompete. München (Germany): JJ Lentner'sche Buchhandlung; 1870.)

Within the cartilaginous portion of the eustachian tube, there is mucosa-associated lymphatic tissue.[15] Lymphatic tissue of the nasopharynx, on the other hand, does not extend into the tube.[16]

Ligaments and Fasciae

Between the tubal cartilage and the skull base there is a system of superior tubal ligaments.[17] It consists of the medial and the lateral tubal suspensory ligament, which are divided by a thin layer of fat tissue, the so-called medial Ostmann fat pad.[4] These ligaments are tangentially connected to the medial and the lateral lamina of the cartilage. In a 3-dimensional (3D) view, these ligaments resemble a fibrous plate rather than a ligament. They arise from the temporal as well as the sphenoid bone. The most constant structure is the lateral suspensory ligament that is connected to the lateral lamina. This lateral suspensory ligament partially connects to the tendinous fibers of the lateral layer of the tensor veli palatini muscle.[4]

There are 2 fasciae that cover the medial and the lateral surface of the tensor veli palatini muscle. Laterally, there is the Weber-Liel fascia, which separates the tensor veli palatine muscle from the medial pterygoid muscle. Medially, there is a fascia that runs from the lateral lamina of the tubal cartilage along the lateral surface of the so-called lateral Ostmann fat pad to the salpingopharyngeal fascia, which is also called the von Tröltsch fascia.

Thus, the lateral suspensory ligaments, the lateral lamina of the cartilage, as well as the Ostmann fat pad constitute a common functional unit.

Membranous Wall

Opposite to the tubal cartilage, there is the so-called membranous wall of the eustachian tube. This wall mainly consists of the tensor veli palatini muscle and of the levator veli palatini muscle; Rüdinger called it "muscular wall."[7] Nevertheless, there is a third anatomic compartment, which contributes to the muscular function: the lateral Ostmann fat pad. That is why the term "membranous wall" is more common. Additional to the constant "lateral Ostmann fat pad" between the lateral lamina and the lateral wall of the eustachian tube, other fatty tissue is found in characteristic locations, of which the medial Ostmann fat pad between the tubal suspensory ligaments is the most important.

The maximum average thickness of the lateral Ostmann fat pad is 2.4 mm. The position of this maximum is found about 20 mm proximal to the pharyngeal orifice. From this point, the Ostmann fat pad gradually decreases toward both orifices. Rüdinger[7] estimated the average thickness of the lateral tubal wall, consisting of its mucous membrane and the Ostmann fat pad, to be 2 mm. According to Rüdinger, this fat pad does not correlate to the body weight. During childhood and adolescence, the thickness of Ostmann fat pad corresponds to its thickness in adults.[18] However, its height increases during postnatal life, causing a growth in volume. This volume decreases again with advanced age.[19] This physiologic decrease does not necessarily cause a patulous eustachian tube.

There are 2 different roles of the lateral Ostmann fat pad:

- First, the static pressure of the fat pad supports the passive closure of the eustachian tube after contraction of the tensor veli palatini muscle.[4] This closing effect helps to prevent the ascension of fluids and acoustic noise from the nasopharynx toward the middle ear. This effect is nondirectional: at the same time the fat pad may prevent the evacuation of the middle ear due to a rapid decrease of nasopharyngeal pressure as postulated by the sniff theory.[20]
- Second, the fat pad serves as a hypomochlion for the lateral layer of the tensor veli palatini muscle.[21] It transfers the pressure of the almost isometric contraction of the muscle to the lower portion of the eustachian tube. Hence, the lateral Ostmann fat pad limits the eustachian tube opening to the Rüdinger safety canal.

Muscles

Although both the tensor and the levator veli palatini muscles are a part of the membranous wall of the eustachian tube, the muscles need to be depicted separately. **Fig. 3** shows a methanal-fixated anatomic specimen of the muscles surrounding the eustachian tube.

Four muscles around the eustachian tube contribute to its function: the tensor and levator veli palatini muscles, the medial pterygoid muscle, and the salpingopharyngeal muscle, albeit its respective impact still is a matter of discussion.[22]

Tensor veli palatini muscle

Today most investigators consider the tensor veli palatini muscle the essential eustachian tube muscle.[10] It is activated by swallowing and by yawning. Its motoric innervation belongs to the mandibular nerve. Its fibers originate from the sphenoid spine, the scaphoid fossa, and the lateral lamina of the tubal cartilage, the posterior half of the membranous tubal wall, and the salpingopharyngeal fascia.[16,23] The muscle forms an inverse triangle, which is located in a skull base niche.[22] The tensor consists of a

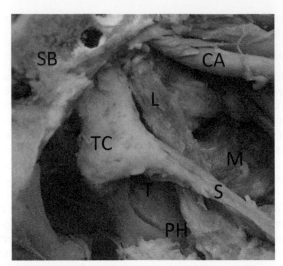

Fig. 3. Muscles contributing to the eustachian tube function. CA, carotid artery; L, levator veli palatini muscle; M, medial pterygoid muscle; PH, pterygoid hamulus; S, salpingopharyngeal muscle; SB, skull base; T, tensor veli palatini muscle; TC, tubal cartilage.

lateral layer originating from the skull base and a medial layer arising from the lateral lamina of the tubal cartilage. Both layers can be partly but not entirely separated by fatty tissue.[10] The lateral layer pulls from the skull base to a small tendon going around the pterygoid hamulus and spreading into the aponeurosis of the soft palate.[4] Between the tendon and the hamulus there is a small bursa. The medial layer of the tensor is situated between the lateral lamina of the tubal cartilage and the medial lamina of the pterygoid process. The function of the tensor veli palatini muscle is complex[22,24] for the 2 following reasons:

- Apart from the bursa at the pterygoid hamulus, the contraction of both layers is completely isometric, meaning that the muscular function depends on hypomochlia, which influence its force vectors. **Fig. 4** shows the force vectors influencing the tensor veli palatini muscle and the tubal cartilage.
- Both layers have dissimilar effects on eustachian tube function: whereas contraction of the medial layer opens the eustachian tube by lateralization of the lateral lamina of the cartilage (see **Fig. 4**, force vector 3), the lateral layer compresses the lower portion of the tube, the membranous wall. Thus, the medial layer supports ventilation, and the lateral layer supports drainage and protection.

There are 3 hypomochlia influencing the tensor veli palatini muscle:

- The pterygoid hamulus[25]
- The lateral Ostmann fat pad[21] (see **Fig. 4**: force vector 2)
- The medial pterygoid muscle[22]

Medial pterygoid muscle

The medial pterygoid muscle is a chewing muscle, which closes the mouth and helps in protruding the mandibula. Like the tensor veli palatini muscle, its innervation arises from the mandibular nerve. According to Leuwer and colleagues,[22] the medial pterygoid muscle is an elastic hypomochlion of the tensor. Its contraction causes a posteromedial movement of the tensor toward the cartilage, increasing the tubal opening

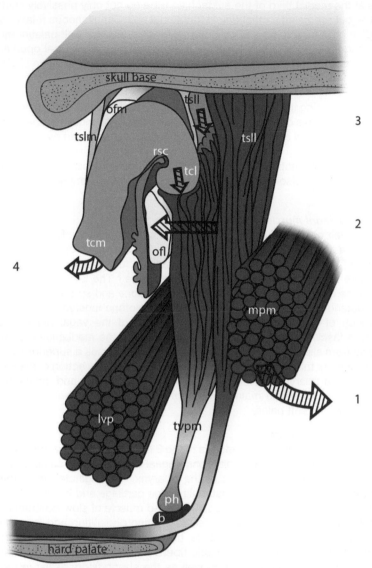

Fig. 4. Pseudo-3D illustration of the eustachian tube showing the force vectors influencing the eustachian tube function. (1) Anterolateral rotation of the medial pterygoid muscle during relaxation, decreasing the tubal opening pressure. (2) Pressure of the lateral layer of the tensor veli palatini muscle on Ostmann fat pad and auxiliary gap. (3) Laterocaudal traction of the lateral lamina of the tubal cartilage and tubal suspensory ligaments. (4) Mediocranial rotation of the medial lamina of the tubal cartilage.

pressure. Inversely, the opening of the eustachian tube is facilitated by the relaxation of the medial pterygoid due to an anterolateral movement of the tensor while opening the mouth (see **Fig. 4**, force vector 1). As described earlier, between the tensor veli palatini muscle and the medial pterygoid muscle there is the Weber-Liel fascia. On both sides of this fascia, Wenzel[26] found fibromuscular interconnections. Thus, both muscles at the medial third of the eustachian tube do not only passively shift against each other but represent a mechanical functional unit. Simultaneous relaxation of the medial pterygoid muscle as well as contraction of the tensor veli palatini muscle by yawning can be used as a maneuver for the physiologic active tubal opening during external pressure changes, such as the landing of an airplane ("Eppendorf manoeuver"[27]).

Also, according to Bylander[28] and Magnuson,[29] the eustachian tube opening can be facilitated by opening the mouth alone. These fibromuscular interconnections can give an explanation for this observation. On the other hand, the function of the tensor muscle can be understood as a passive diaphragm, actively regulated by the medial pterygoid muscle.

Morphological or functional alterations of the medial pterygoid muscle, for example, in craniomandibular disorders, may change the muscular compliance of the eustachian tube.

Levator veli palatini muscle

The levator veli palatini muscle is located inferolateral to the inferior margin of the medial lamina of the eustachian tube cartilage.[30] Although it is close to the medial lamina, crossing the longitudinal axis of the eustachian tube at the so-called tubal incisure,[16] there is no direct attachment to the cartilage.[1] The levator originates at the lower surface of the petrous part of the temporal bone and spreads out into the soft palate, posteriorly to the pterygoid hamulus. Its motoric innervation is provided by each branch of the glossopharyngeal as well as of the vagal nerve.[31] Bryant[23] described a fascial attachment to the inferior edge of the medial lamina preventing the muscle from slipping off the cartilage. The levator causes a superior-medial rotation of the anterior tubal cartilage, thus assisting to a pumping action of the eustachian tube toward the pharyngeal orifice. According to Finkelstein and colleagues[32] and based on clinical data, the main function of the levator muscle is restricted to the competence of the soft palate.

Salpingopharyngeal muscle

The salpingopharyngeal muscle belongs to the 3 internal longitudinal pharyngeal muscles (stylopharyngeal muscle, palatopharyngeal muscle, and salpingopharyngeal muscle),[33] which are the elevators of the pharynx.[34] It originates from the inferior edge of the medial lamina of the eustachian tube cartilage and inserts into the longitudinal fibers of the pharynx. The muscle is a red muscle of slow contraction speed, adapted for sustained contraction. It relaxes during deglutition and is active at rest with the mouth shut.[35] Within the muscle, there are bundles of muscle fibers as well as groups of elastic fibers. These elastic fibers are also attached to the floor of the eustachian tube. Thus, the muscle as well as the elastic fibers assist in the closure of the anterior tube. Hence, its action is antagonistic to the tensor and levator veli palatini muscles. **Fig. 4** shows that there is a rolling force vector from the medial lamina of the eustachian tube cartilage (see **Fig. 4**, force vector 4). This force vector is caused by the contraction of the medial layer of the tensor veli palatini muscle. Considering this force vector, the salpingopharyngeal muscle gives the impression of an anchor chain controlling the position of the medial lamina and keeping the pharyngeal orifice of the eustachian tube in position.

REFFRENCES

1. Pahnke J. Beiträge zur Klinischen Anatomie der Tuba Auditiva. Würzburg (Germany): Medizinische Habilitationsschrift; 1991.

2. Dinc AE, Damar M, Ugur MB, et al. Do the angle and length of the Eustachian tube influence the development of chronic otitis media? Laryngoscope 2015; 125:2187–92.

3. Proctor B. Embryology and anatomy of the Eustachian tube. Arch Otolaryngol 1967;86:503–14.

4. Zöllner F. Anatomie, Physiologie, Pathologie und Klinik der Ohrtrompete und ihre Diagnostisch-Therapeutischen Beziehungen zu allen Nachbarschafterkrankungen. In: Zange J, editor. Hals-, Nasen-, Ohrenheilkunde der Gegenwart und ihre Grenzgebiete. Berlin: Springer; 1942. p. 1–213.

5. Warwick R, Williams PL. Gray's anatomy. Edinburgh (United Kingdom): Longman; 1973.

6. Luntz M, Pitashny R, Sadé J. Cartilage in the bony portion of the Eustachian tube. In: Sadé J, editor. Basic aspects of the Eustachian tube and middle ear diseases. Amsterdam: Kugler and Ghedini; 1991. p. 17–22.

7. Rüdinger N. Vergleichende Anatomie und Histologie der Ohrtrompete. München (Germany): JJ Lentneŕsche Buchhandlung; 1870.

8. Oshima T, Kikuchi T, Hori Y, et al. Magnetic resonance imaging of the eustachian tube cartilage. Acta Otolaryngol 2008;128:510–4.

9. Bluestone CD. Eustachian tube: structure, function, role in otitis media. Hamilton (Canada): BC Decker; 2005.

10. Pahnke J. Morphology, function, and clinical aspects of the Eustachian tube. In: Jahnke K, editor. Middle ear surgery. Thieme: Stuttgart; 2004. p. 1–22.

11. Matsune S, Sando I, Takahashi H. Elastin at the hinge portion of the Eustachian tube cartilage in specimens from normal subjects and those with cleft palate. Ann Otol Rhinol Laryngol 1992;101:163–7.

12. Schilder AGM, Bhutta MF, Butler CC, et al. Eustachian tube dysfunction: consensus statement on definition, types, clinical presentation and diagnosis. Clin Otolaryngol 2015;40:407–11.

13. Sando I, Takahashi H, Matsune S, et al. Localization of function in the Eustachian tube: a hypothesis. Ann Otol Rhinol Laryngol 1994;103:311–4.

14. Ozturk K, Snyderman CH, Sando I. Do mucosal folds in the eustachian tube function as microturbinates? Laryngoscope 2011;212:821–4.

15. Matsune S, Takahashi H, Sando I. Mucosa-associated lymphoid tissue in middle ear and Eustachian tube in children. Int J Pediatr Otorhinolaryngol 1996;34: 229–36.

16. Aschan G. The anatomy of the Eustachian tube with regard to its function. Acta Soc Med Ups 1955;60:131–49.

17. Proctor B. Anatomy of the Eustachian tube. Arch Otolaryngol 1973;97:2–9.

18. Aoki H, Sando I, Takahashi H. Anatomic relationships between Ostmann's fatty tissue and Eustachian tube. Ann Otol Rhinol Laryngol 1994;103:211–4.

19. Amoodi H, Bance M, Thamboo A. Magnetic resonance imaging illustrating change in the Ostmann fat pad with age. J Otolaryngol Head Neck Surg 2010; 39:440–1.

20. Magnuson B. Tubal opening and closing ability in unilateral middle ear disease. Am J Otolaryngol 1981;2:199–209.

21. Pahnke J, Hoppe F, Hofmann E, et al. Funktionelle Anatomie des Ostmannschen Fettkörpers. HNO 1990;47:428.

22. Leuwer R, Schubert R, Kucinski T, et al. The muscular compliance of the auditory tube: a model-based survey. Laryngoscope 2002;112:1791–5.

23. Bryant WS. The Eustachian tube, its anatomy and its movement: with a description of the cartilages, muscles, fasciae, and the fossa of Rosenmüller. Med Rec 1907;71:931–4.
24. Guild SR. Elastic tissue of the Eustachian tube. Ann Otol Rhinol Laryngol 1956;64:537–43.
25. Sehhati-Chafai-Leuwer S, Wenzel S, Bschorer R, et al. Pathophysiology of the Eustachian tube—relevant new aspects for the head and neck surgeon. J Craniomaxillofac Surg 2006;34:351–4.
26. Wenzel S. Die Verschlussinsuffizienz der Tuba Auditiva—Neue Aspekte zur Pathogenese, Diagnostik und Therapie von Mittelohrprotektionsstörungen. Hamburg (Germany): Habilitationsschrift; 2004.
27. Leuwer R, Schubert R, Wenzel S, et al. New aspects of the mechanics of the auditory tube. HNO 2003;51:431–8.
28. Bylander A. Comparison of eustachian tube function in children and adults with normal ear. Ann Otol Rhinol Laryngol 1980;89(Suppl 68):20–4.
29. Magnuson B. On the origin of the high negative pressure in the middle ear space. Am J Otolaryngol 1981;2:1–12.
30. Ishijima K, Sando I, Balaban CD, et al. Functional anatomy of the levator veli palatine muscle and tensor veli palatine muscle in association with Eustachian tube cartilage. Ann Otol Rhinol Laryngol 2002;111:530–53.
31. Shimokawa T, Yi SQ, Izumi A, et al. An anatomical study of the levator veli palatini and superior constrictor with special reference to their nerve supply. Surg Radiol Anat 2004;26:100–5.
32. Finkelstein Y, Talmi YP, Nachmani A, et al. Pathology of levator veli palatini muscle and Eustachian tube. In: Conference of the Eustachian tube and middle ear diseases. Geneva, October 26-29, 1989.
33. Choi DY, Bae JH, Youn KH, et al. Anatomical considerations of the longitudinal pharyngeal muscles in relation to their function on the internal surface of pharynx. Dysphagia 2014;29:722–30.
34. Schünke M, Schulte E, Schumacher U. Prometheus Kopf-, Hals- und Neuroanatomie: Lernatlas Anatomie. Thieme: Stuttgart; 2012.
35. Guindi GM, Charia KKC. A reappraisal of the salpingo-pharyngeus muscle. Arch Otorhinolaryngol 1980;229:135–41.

Endoscopic Anatomy of the Protympanum

Nicholas Jufas, MBBS, MS, FRACS[a,b,c], Daniele Marchioni, MD[d],
Muaaz Tarabichi, MD[e], Nirmal Patel, MBBS, MS, FRACS[a,b,c],*

KEYWORDS

- Endoscopic ear surgery • Protympanum • Surgical anatomy • Tensor tympani
- Carotid artery • Protiniculum

KEY POINTS

- The protympanum, a final common pathway between the tympanic cavity and external environment, is gaining relevance due to the ease and completeness of visualization with angled endoscopes.
- Two primary conformations are described, quadrangular and triangular, and new anatomic structures such as the protiniculum, subtensor recess (SbTR), caroticocochlear recess, and protympanic spine are defined.
- The SbTR, an area of pneumatization inferomedial to the tensor tympani canal (TC) is shown to have 3 conformations: flat TC/absent SbTr (A), raised TC/shallow SbTR (B), and raised TC/deep SbTR (C).
- The protiniculum, a consistent bony ridge from the promontory to the lateral wall demarcating the transition between the hypotympanum and protympanum, is shown to have 3 conformations: ridge (A), bridge (B), and absent (C).
- Surgical relevance of the protympanum is described with respect to ventilation, cholesteatoma, cerebrospinal fluid leak, otic neuralgia, and balloon dilatation of the eustachian tube.

 Video content accompanies this article at http://www.oto.theclinics.com.

INTRODUCTION

The protympanum, or bony portion of the eustachian tube (ET), is a middle ear space that lies anterior to the mesotympanum. The space is also confluent with the epitympanum superiorly, hypotympanum inferiorly, and the cartilaginous ET anteriorly.

No disclosures.
[a] Kolling Deafness Research Centre, University of Sydney and Macquarie University, Sydney, Australia; [b] Discipline of Surgery, Sydney Medical School, University of Sydney, Sydney, Australia; [c] Sydney Endoscopic Ear Surgery (SEES) Research Group, Sydney, Australia; [d] Otolaryngology Department, University Hospital of Verona, Piazzale Aristide Stefani, 37122, Verona, Italy; [e] ENT Department, American Hospital Dubai, 19th St, Oud Metha Rd, Dubai, United Arab Emirates
* Corresponding author. Suite A12, 24-32 Lexington Drive, Bella Vista, New South Wales 2153, Australia.
E-mail address: nirmal.p.patel@gmail.com

Otolaryngol Clin N Am 49 (2016) 1107–1119
http://dx.doi.org/10.1016/j.otc.2016.05.009
0030-6665/16/$ – see front matter © 2016 Elsevier Inc. All rights reserved.

The protympanum has been infrequently examined in the past due to its difficulty to view using the operating microscope.[1] However, the area is now gaining relevance with endoscopic ear surgery because it can easily be seen with angled scopes. With surgery moving toward evaluation and restoration of ventilation pathways,[2] the protympanum serves as the final common pathway between the tympanic cavity and external environment, drawing comparisons to the ventilatory function of the larynx in the airway.[3]

EMBRYOLOGY

True ossification of the protympanum only commences at the 18th fetal week because of its dependence on the bone growth of the otic capsule.[4] Earlier studies reported a contribution to protympanum development from the tympanic part of the temporal bone,[5] while more recent studies point to development solely from the petrous part of the temporal bone.[4]

From the 21st fetal week, 2 bony laminae develop around the carotid artery, eventually forming the carotid canal. The superior lamina is better developed, forming 2 prolongations: a superior, which is longer and connects to the tympanic annulus posteriorly, forming the lateral wall of the protympanum; and an inferior prolongation, which is shorter and forms the lateral wall of the carotid canal. Similarly, from the 23rd fetal week, the canal for the tensor tympani muscle forms from superior and inferior laminae. In addition, the tegmen tympani and promontory help to form the superior and medial walls of the protympanum, respectively.[4]

BOUNDARIES

The boundaries of the protympanum had been previously defined as the most anterior extent of horizontal and vertical tangents through the margins of the osseous tympanic ring.[6] The boundaries can now be defined more clearly with angled endoscopes (**Fig. 1**).

- *Superior*: tegmen tympani and entire tensor tympani canal, merging posteriorly with and including the supratubal recess if present, with the boundary defined here by the tensor fold;
- *Inferior*: from the protiniculum (an oblique bony ridge demarcating the transition from hypotympanum) posteriorly, extending anteriorly with the possible presence of protympanic air cells, an anterior extension of the hypotympanic cell complex;
- *Anterior*: confluent with the junctional and then cartilaginous portion of the ET;
- *Posterior*: confluent with the mesotympanum;
- *Medial*: lateral wall of the carotid canal, extending from the caroticocochlear recess anteriorly, with caroticotympanic vessels and nerves including anterior branches from Jacobson's (tympanic branch of glossopharyngeal) nerve. More anteriorly, variations of false passages occur depending on pneumatization patterns.
- *Lateral*: bony wall separating the space from the mandibular fossa and extending to the anterior annulus, from the level of the protiniculum inferiorly to the anterior limit of the notch of Rivinus at the anterior tympanic spine.

Superior Boundary

The predominant feature of the superior boundary is tensor tympani canal. The region superolateral to the tensor canal forms the supratubal recess. The supratubal recess has a variable size or is absent, depending on the orientation of the tensor tympani fold. Önal and colleagues[7] described 2 principal configurations of the anterior epitympanic space: type I (83%) consists of an oblique (and occasionally vertical) tensor

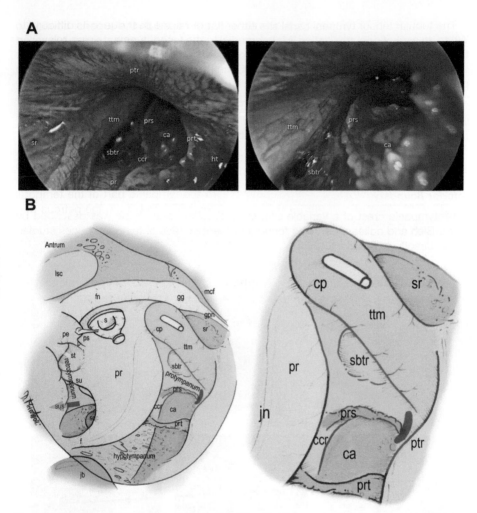

Fig. 1. (*A*) Endoscopic view of protympanum in the right ear with 30° endoscope angled anteriorly. (*Left*) View just after passing beyond the anterior annulus of the tympanic membrane. (*Right*) View obtained by inserting endoscope deeper to visualize the lumen of the ET (*asterisk*). (*B*) Schematic drawing of middle ear (*left*), including the protympanum, its anatomic boundaries, and important structures contained within. Detailed view of protympanum (*right*). ca, carotid artery; ccr, caroticocochlear recess; cp, cochleariform process; f, finiculus; fn, facial nerve; gg, geniculate ganglion; gpn, greater superficial petrosal nerve; ht, hypotympanum; jb, jugular bulb; jn, Jacobson's nerve; lsc, lateral semicircular canal; mcf, middle cranial fossa; p, ponticulus; pe, pyramidal eminence; pr, promontory; prs, protympanic spine; prt, protiniculum; ps, posterior sinus; ptr, pretympanic recess; s, stapes; sbtr, subtensor recess; sr, supratubal recess; st, sinus tympani; su, subiculum; sus, sinus subtympanicus; ttm, tensor tympani muscle.

tympani fold that creates a smaller anterior epitympanic space and the presence of a supratubal recess; type II (17%) consists of a more horizontally placed tensor fold, which does not allow for the presence of a supratubal recess. The superior boundary of the supratubal recess (if present) is the tensor fold, which is occasionally incomplete.

The tubular tensor tympani canal sits either flat or raised on the superior boundary. When an area of pneumatization is inferomedial to the tensor tympani canal, it is called the subtensor recess (SbTR). To keep endoscopic anatomic nomenclature consistent with previous descriptions of the retrotympanum,[8] there are 3 apparent conformations possible based on the depth of the SbTR when present (**Fig. 2**):

- *Type A*: Flat tensor canal, absent SbTR;
- *Type B*: Raised tensor canal, shallow SbTR, easily visible fundus;
- *Type C*: Raised tensor canal, deep SbTR, difficult to see limits of fundus.

Demarcation between a type B and type C SbTR is when the fundus of the SbTR extends superior to the midpoint of the tensor tympani canal.

Inferior Boundary

A protympanic crest of a variable site, size, direction, and shape was described by Abou-Bieh and colleagues,[9] who found it present in 79% of temporal bones studied either directly or radiologically.

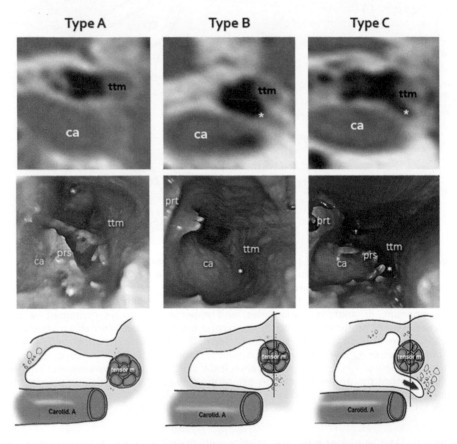

Fig. 2. Demonstration of the possible conformations of the SbTR (*asterisk*), with computed tomographic (*top*) endoscopic (*middle*), and schematic (*bottom*) views of left ears corresponding to the 3 types. Type A: flat tensor canal, absent SbTR; type B: raised tensor canal, shallow SbTR, easily visible fundus; type C: raised tensor canal, deep SbTR, difficult to see limits of fundus.

In temporal bones studied endoscopically by the authors, a bony ridge was commonly found extending from the promontory on the medial wall, across the inferior wall and merging with the lateral wall. The medial aspect of the ridge consistently marked the end of the most anterior hypotympanic air cell, and thus, the start of the protympanum.

This bony ridge has therefore been named the protiniculum (from the Latin *protinus*: forward, farther on), in keeping with previously described nomenclature of promontorial bony ridges in the middle ear.[10] The protiniculum has 3 conformations (**Fig. 3**):

- *Type A*: Ridge, with no air cells passing medially;
- *Type B*: Bridge, with hypotympanic air cells extending inferiorly into the protympanum;
- *Type C*: Absent, no discernible protiniculum, the hypotympanum fusing with the protympanum.

Anterior Boundary

The anterior boundary of the protympanum is a transition point into the junctional and then cartilaginous portions of the ET. It can be reliably found by following the junction of the superior and lateral walls of the epitympanum anteriorly, with the tensor tympani muscle medially, which consistently seems to ensure that false passages are not entered.

The exact point of transition at the anterior boundary however is difficult to define endoscopically. As the protympanum continues toward the anterior boundary, the tensor tympani muscle rotates 90° around the superior wall in a clockwise (right) or counterclockwise (left) fashion, taking it from a medial to a lateral position, consistent with the theory that the tensor veli palatini muscle, which attaches to the entire lateral cartilaginous portion of the ET, forms a functional unit with the tensor tympani.[11]

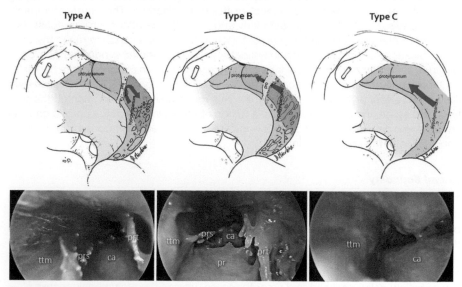

Fig. 3. Demonstration of the possible conformations of the protiniculum with schematic (*top*) and endoscopic (*bottom*) views of right ears corresponding to the 3 types. Type A: ridge, with no air cells passing medially; type B: bridge, with hypotympanic air cells extending inferiorly into the protympanum; type C: absent, no discernible protiniculum, the hypotympanum fusing with the protympanum.

Medial and Posterior Boundary

In a series of 1000 formalin-fixed temporal bones, carotid canal dehiscence on the medial wall of the protympanum has been identified in up to 7.7% of temporal bones and was more common in patients younger than 2 years and older than 40 years.[12] The dehiscence generally arises from failure of the laminae to fuse congenitally,[4] but microdehiscences may be secondary to bony resorption later in life.[12] In a smaller series of 150 temporal bones, the mean thickness of the thinnest bone overlying the carotid artery was 1.5 mm (range 0–3 mm), and bulging of the carotid artery into the protympanum was barely indicated in 31%, moderately noticeable in 56%, and markedly noticeable in 13%.[13]

Jacobson's nerve or the tympanic branch of the glossopharyngeal nerve is a bundle of predominantly secretomotor and sensory fibers. The nerve leaves the inferior ganglion above the jugular foramen and traverses the inferior tympanic canaliculus to enter the middle ear either through or just anterior to the finiculus. The first branches of the tympanic nerve tend to occur above the round window.[14] The nerve traverses anteromedially to form the posterior boundary of the protympanum.

The tympanic nerve is the main contributing nerve to the tympanic plexus, which lies on the promontory. The plexus is usually submucosal; however, the nerves may lie deeper and groove the bone and rarely are embedded in the bone of the promontory.[15] The tympanic nerve provides sensation to the protympanum and ET as well delivers parasympathetic fibers that arise in the inferior salivary nucleus to the same region. The nerve exits the middle ear space, medial to the tensor tympani tendon, and becomes the lesser superficial petrosal nerve carrying the visceral motor parasympathetic fibers from the tympanic plexus to the parotid gland via the otic ganglion. Further parasympathetic supply reaches the tympanic plexus via the nervus intermedius and the facial nerve at the geniculate ganglion.

The caroticotympanic nerves and arteries exit through channels in the bone overlying the carotid canal on the medial aspect of the protympanum. The caroticotympanic nerves carry sympathetic fibers posteriorly and cross the caroticocochlear recess, between the anterior aspect of the promontory and the carotid canal, to reach the tympanic plexus. Postganglionic oculosympathetic palsy (Horner syndrome) has been reported secondary to middle ear infections, likely through an effect on these nerves.[16]

Occasionally, a rough spine composed of either bony ridges or spicules is seen over the carotid artery prominence (see **Fig. 1**). This rough spine has been named the protympanic spine and is likely related to a fusion of the 2 laminae of the carotid canal in embryologic development. If so, it may indicate a decreased likelihood of carotid canal dehiscence in the protympanum.

Lateral Boundary

The lateral lamina separates the protympanum from the mandibular fossa. The lamina is the only boundary of the protympanum that has some contribution from the tympanic part of the temporal bone on the posterior aspect.[4] It is more commonly convex toward the lumen, but may also be concave. A convex conformation appears to result in a narrower lumen and may obstruct view of the anterior boundary, even when using an angled endoscope. In the posterior aspect of the lateral lamina, just medial to the annular sulcus lies a shallow, relatively short and smooth recess, named the pretympanic recess.[17]

Superolaterally is the opening of the petrotympanic (Glaserian) fissure, between the bony annulus of the tympanic and petrous parts of the temporal bone, and containing the anterior malleolar ligament (AML) and discomalleolar ligaments (DML), anterior tympanic artery, and chorda tympani nerve.[18] The AML extends from the neck of the malleus, traverses the fissure, attaches to the capsule of the temporomandibular joint, and is closely associated with the smaller DML.[19] The anterior tympanic artery arises from the first (mandibular) part of the maxillary artery, traverses the fissure, and gives rise to a superior, posterior, and ossicular branch.[20] The chorda tympani nerve exits the middle ear medial to the AML and through the petrotympanic fissure in the separate anterior chordal canal, also known as the iter chordae anterius, Civinini canal, or Huguier canal,[21] traveling superolateral to the ET to reach the lingual nerve.[17] Dehiscence of the anterior chordal canal as well as demonstrated connections between the AML/DML and sphenomandibular ligament may allow for putative anatomic explanation of otomandibular (Costen) syndrome.[18,22]

CONFORMATIONS

The protympanic space has 2 main conformations[5]:

- Quadrangular
- Triangular

The conformational shape is interpreted from the anteriorly facing 30° endoscopic appearance. From this view, a 2-dimensional plane perpendicular to the long axis of ET, passing through the carotid prominence and lateral wall just anterior to the junction with the pretympanic space, is projected.

Demarcation between the 2 types is based on whether the inferior wall is more (quadrangular) or less (triangular) than half the length of the superior wall in equivalent transverse dimension. An irregular shape has also been described, but is likely due to the presence of air cells or taken in a plane that is oblique to that described above. Demarcation between the 2 types also appears to correlate well with computed tomography reconstructions in the same 2-dimensional perpendicular plane (**Fig. 4**).

The quadrangular shape (previously referred to as rectangular) is more common and generally has a carotid artery that is further removed from the tympanic opening of the lumen. A triangular shape forms when the medial and lateral walls merge inferiorly, occasionally obliterating the inferior wall completely. This conformation appears to be less commonly associated with the presence of air cells and potential for false passages.

A video has been included as a supplement to the text and figures of this article, summarizing the anatomic boundaries of the protympanum as well as the conformations of the structures contained therein (Video 1).

NEUROLYMPHOVASCULAR SUPPLY OF THE PROTYMPANUM

The sensory supply of the protympanum is predominantly via the glossopharyngeal nerve (CN IX) and principally Jacobson's nerve.[17] The tubal branch of the tympanic plexus was first described by Ludwig Jacobson in 1818.

Autonomic supply of the area is from the petrosal nerves, Jacobson's nerve, and caroticotympanic branches.[17]

The lymphatics of the region predominantly drain via bony channels and the external auditory canal to the parotid nodes. Accessory drainage occurs via parapharyngeal and retropharyngeal nodes to the upper jugular chain.[17]

Arterial supply to the protympanum is predominantly from anastomoses of the following[20]:

- *The tubal artery*, which branches from the accessory meningeal artery, in turn a branch of the middle meningeal artery from the first (mandibular) portion of the maxillary artery, or more commonly, from the maxillary artery directly;

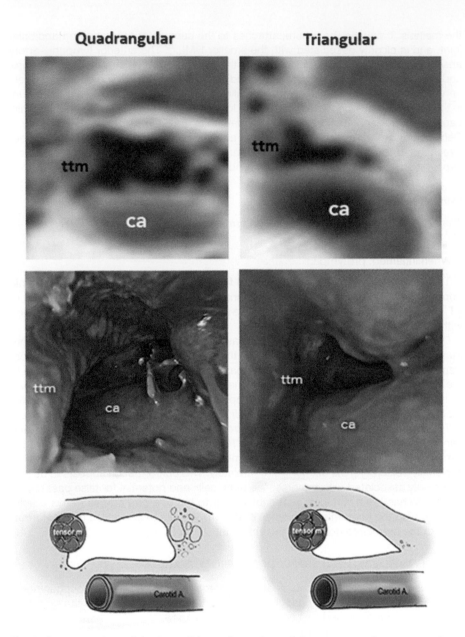

Fig. 4. Demonstration of the 2 possible conformations of the protympanic space, quadrangular and triangular, with computed tomographic (*top*), endoscopic (*middle*), and schematic (*bottom*) views of right ears.

- *Caroticotympanic arteries* (usually a total of 2), which arise from the internal carotid artery and enter the protympanum through bony channels in the caroticocochlear recess;
- *Inferior tympanic artery*, a branch of the ascending pharyngeal artery, in turn a branch of the external carotid artery, enters the middle ear through the inferior

tympanic canaliculus with Jacobson's nerve, then ascends over the promontory in a small groove or canal.

A venous plexus, located along the length of the ET submucosa, drains almost entirely to the pterygoid plexus and via caroticotympanic veins to the paracarotid venous plexus. This plexus may give rise to tubal varices.[17]

MORPHOFUNCTIONAL IMPORTANCE OF THE PROTYMPANUM

Over the promontory and within the protympanum, the mucosa is pseudostratified epithelium. Numerous mucous-secreting and ciliated cells are present, resembling nasal mucosa. The connective tissue here is thicker and denser, and its physiologic function is predominantly mucociliary clearance toward the ET. In contrast, in the posterior mesotympanum and epitympanum, the epithelium is flat with thin, loose connective tissue and no mucous or ciliated cells. This area is devoted to gas exchange, similar to the mastoid mucosa.[23]

When inflamed, protympanic epithelium thickens and may become polypoid. Electron microscopy has demonstrated a decrease in ciliated cells, with collapse of residual cilia and evidence of stagnation with mucous secretion. Mucosal cells contain numerous secretory granules, and there was evidence of polymorphonuclear cells submucousally and bacteria at the mucosal surface.[24]

There appears to be a high prevalence of biofilm formation in both the middle ear and the adenoid bed in chronic otitis media.[25,26] Given its anatomic location, biofilms are likely to be present in the protympanum.

These factors may lead to sequelae such as otitis media with effusion or perforation of the tympanic membrane in the acute setting. In the chronic setting, obstruction leads to a negative pressure in the mesotympanum, facilitating processes such as tympanic membrane retraction and chronic otitis media.[23]

SURGICAL IMPORTANCE OF THE PROTYMPANUM
Final Common Pathway of Ventilation

Considering the morphofunctional importance of the protympanum in the ventilation of the middle ear and mastoid system as well as the development of chronic otitis media, more attention is being paid to disease clearance in this region. The use of 30° and 45° scopes along with angled instruments allows easy access to the boundaries of the protympanum, including the lateral wall for removal of granulation and inflamed mucosa.

Future therapies may investigate the locally targeted application of steroids or other anti-inflammatory mediators to reduce inflammation in this region. Reducing inflammation in this region may in turn lead to a reduction of chronic otitis media or retraction, in an attempt to reduce long-term sequelae.

Cholesteatoma in the Protympanum

The protympanum is a region where cholesteatoma is seldom found, but when present, is often difficult to completely visualize and access. Cholesteatoma in the protympanum is more likely to occur with the following:

- The congenital form of the disease;
- Extensive anterior epitympanic disease with an incomplete tensor fold; or
- Aggressive mesotympanic disease.

Adjunct inspection of the protympanum with a mirror or after drilling of relevant bony landmarks for direct visualization has been recommended in cholesteatoma surgery for many years. The introduction of endoscopes initially allowed adjunct inspection to check for residual disease.[27] More recently, angled endoscopes have been used exclusively to perform surgery in difficult to access areas.[28] In the protympanum, this will allow full and direct visualization to safely remove disease as well as identify previously hidden regions such as false passages, air cells, and the SbTR. An example of protympanic cholesteatoma being fully visualized and completely removed is shown in **Fig. 5**.

With aggressive disease in this region, and with experienced hands, consideration can be given to anterior mobilization of the tensor tympani muscle to reach aggressive disease in the superior and medial walls of the protympanum. Specifically designed instruments, with an appropriate length and angulation, or with a malleable tip, may help to ensure safe and complete disease removal from the protympanum.

Cerebrospinal Fluid Leak

Although the incidence of cerebrospinal fluid leak following lateral skull base surgery has decreased, it remains a reported complication in at least 5% of operative cases.[29] The final common pathway of a transnasal leak is via the protympanum into the nasopharynx. In recalcitrant cases, closure of the ET using transnasal endoscopes to seal the pharyngeal orifice has been reported.[30]

Knowledge of the protympanic spaces and full visualization with an angled endoscope can help the surgeon have confidence in identifying the true ET for safely packing the region. Identifying false passages and pneumatization patterns in the area may help explain leaks that persist after apparent treatment.

Otic Neuralgia

Neurovascular compression of the glossopharyngeal nerve at the route entry zone or variably along its pathway has been postulated to contribute to otic neuralgia. Division

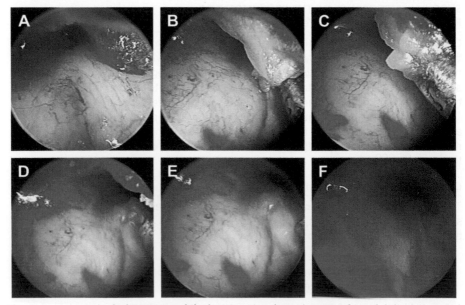

Fig. 5. Protympanic cholesteatoma (*A*), showing time lapse images of careful dissection and removal of disease (*B–E*), with successful clearance of disease (*F*).

of Jacobson's nerve or tympanic neurectomy has been used as a successful treatment of otic neuralgia.[31] A noted additional effect of this procedure is reduction in parasympathetic stimulation on the parotid gland from fibers that travel via the lesser petrosal nerve and synapse in the otic ganglion to supply the parotid through the auriculotemporal nerve. Tympanic neurectomy has therefore been used to ameliorate sequelae of parotid overstimulation such as Frey syndrome, recurrent parotitis, and sialorrhea.[32,33]

When performing the procedure of tympanic neurectomy, attention should be paid to correctly identifying the main trunk of Jacobson's nerve as well as all the branches of the tympanic plexus on the medial wall of the protympanum. It often can groove a channel over the promontory and in up to 20% of cases lies completely encased in a bony canal.[32] Endoscopic visualization of the protympanum and hypotympanum should significantly increase certainty in identification and completeness of division of the main trunk and branches in select cases when this procedure is undertaken.

Surgical Access to the Eustachian Tube

Transtympanic balloon dilatation is being examined as a possible treatment approach in ET dysfunction in failures of transnasal balloon dilatation. Furthermore, this approach to dilatation of the ET may be appropriate in patients who are already undergoing ear surgery for sequelae of ET dysfunction.

Cadaveric work by the authors has demonstrated the feasibility of a balloon dilatation technique using dual endoscopic visualization. No carotid canal fractures were seen in the cohort of 10 heads, and this was verified by 2 surgeons and a board-certified neuroradiologist. Furthermore, efficacy of the dilatation was shown radiologically and via manometry.[34] The use of the endoscope in this technique has fundamentally improved the feasibility and safety in comparison with a previous study, which attempted the same approach with microscopic visualization.[35] Ongoing study is required to clarify the safety of the technique and identify the ideal patient population for treatment.

Further applications of endoscopic protympanic visualisation have been described for managing ET dysfunction. Catheters may be used to gently probe the ET to confirm patency, flush with saline and even instill medical therapy such as topical steroids. Additionally, in cases of patulous ET, a modified catheter inserted transtympanically has been described to shim the ET and reduce severity of symptoms such as autophony.[36]

SUPPLEMENTARY DATA

Supplementary data related to this article can be found at http://dx.doi.org/10.1016/j.otc.2016.05.009.

REFERENCES

1. Thomassin JM, Inedjian JM, Rud C, et al. Otoendoscopy: application in the middle ear surgery. Rev Laryngol Otol Rhinol (Bord) 1990;111(5):475–7 [in French].
2. Marchioni D, Mattioli F, Alicandri-Ciufelli M, et al. Endoscopic evaluation of middle ear ventilation route blockage. Am J Otolaryngol 2010;31(6):453–66.
3. Bluestone CD, Bluestone MB. Eustachian tube. Structure, function, role in otitis media. Shelton (CT): PMPH-USA; 2005. p. 62.
4. Tóth M, Medvegy T, Moser G, et al. Development of the protympanum. Ann Anat 2006;188(3):267–73.

5. Djerić D, Savić D. Anatomical variations and relations of the bony portion of the eustachian tube. Acta Otolaryngol 1985;99(5–6):543–50.

6. Nadol JB, McKenna MJ. Surgery of the ear and temporal bone. Philadelphia (PA): Lippincott Williams & Wilkins; 2005. p. 125.

7. Önal K, van Haastert RM, Grote JJ. Structural variations of the supratubal recess: the anterior epitympanic space. Otol Neurotol 1997;18(3):317.

8. Marchioni D, Mattioli F, Alicandri-Ciufelli M, et al. Transcanal endoscopic approach to the sinus tympani: a clinical report. Otol Neurotol 2009;30(6):758–65.

9. Abou-Bieh AA, Al-Abdulhadi K, Al-Tubaikh J, et al. The protympanic crest. Otolaryngol Head Neck Surg 2009;141(3):92.

10. Marchioni D, Alicandri-Ciufelli M, Piccinini A, et al. Inferior retrotympanum revisited: an endoscopic anatomic study. Laryngoscope 2010;120(9):1880–6.

11. Kierner AC, Mayer R, Kirschhofer von K. Do the tensor tympani and tensor veli palatini muscles of man form a functional unit? A histochemical investigation of their putative connections. Hear Res 2002;165(1–2):48–52.

12. Moreano EH, Paparella MM, Zelterman D, et al. Prevalence of carotid canal dehiscence in the human middle ear: a report of 1000 temporal bones. Laryngoscope 1994;104(5 Pt 1):612–8.

13. Savić D, Djerić D. Anatomical variations and relations in the medial wall of the bony portion of the eustachian tube. Acta Otolaryngol 1985;99(5–6):551–6.

14. Donaldson I. Surgical anatomy of the tympanic nerve. J Laryngol Otol 1980;94(2): 163–8.

15. Rosen S. The tympanic plexus: an anatomic study. Arch Otolaryngol 1950;52(1): 15–8.

16. Spector RH. Postganglionic horner syndrome in three patients with coincident middle ear infection. J Neuroophthalmol 2008;28(3):182–5.

17. Proctor B. Embryology and anatomy of the eustachian tube. Arch Otolaryngol 1967;86(5):503–14.

18. Tóth M, Moser G, Patonay L, et al. Development of the anterior chordal canal. Ann Anat 2006;188(1):7–11.

19. Rodríguez-Vázquez JF, Mérida-Velasco JR, Mérida-Velasco JA, et al. Anatomical considerations on the discomalleolar ligament. J Anat 1998;192(Pt 4):617–21.

20. Merchant SN, Nadol JB. Schuknecht's pathology of the ear. Shelton (CT): PMPH-USA; 2010. p. 61.

21. Mudry A. Glaser fissure, Huguier canal, and Civinini canal: a confused eponymical imbroglio. Otol Neurotol 2015;36(6):1115–20.

22. Eckerdal O. The petrotympanic fissure: a link connecting the tympanic cavity and the temporomandibular joint. Cranio 1991;9(1):15–22.

23. Ars B, Ars-Piret NM. Morphofunctional partition of the middle ear cleft. Mediterr J Otol 2007;3:31–9.

24. Chao W-Y, Chang S-J. Ultrastructure of eustachian tube mucosa in chronic otitis media with cholesteatoma. Am J Otolaryngol 1996;17(3):161–6.

25. Saafan ME, Ibrahim WS, Tomoum MO. Role of adenoid biofilm in chronic otitis media with effusion in children. Eur Arch Otorhinolaryngol 2013;270(9):2417–25.

26. Homøe P, Bjarnsholt T, Wessman M, et al. Morphological evidence of biofilm formation in Greenlanders with chronic suppurative otitis media. Eur Arch Otorhinolaryngol 2009;266(10):1533–8.

27. Thomassin JM, Korchia D, Doris JMD. Endoscopic-guided otosurgery in the prevention of residual cholesteatomas. Laryngoscope 1993;103(8):939–43.

28. Presutti L, Gioacchini FM, Alicandri-Ciufelli M, et al. Results of endoscopic middle ear surgery for cholesteatoma treatment: a systematic review. Acta Otorhinolaryngol Ital 2014;34(3):153–7.
29. Fishman AJ, Marrinan MS, Golfinos JG, et al. Prevention and management of cerebrospinal fluid leak following vestibular schwannoma surgery. Laryngoscope 2004;114(3):501–5.
30. Kwartler JA, Schulder M, Baredes S, et al. Endoscopic closure of the eustachian tube for repair of cerebrospinal fluid leak. Otol Neurotol 1996;17(3):470.
31. Cook JA, Irving RM. Role of tympanic neurectomy in otalgia. J Laryngol Otol 1990;104(02):114–7.
32. Golding-Wood PH. Tympanic neurectomy. J Laryngol Otol 1962;76(09):683–93.
33. Friedman WH, Swerdlow RS, Pomarico JM. Tympanic neurectomy: a review and an additional indication for this procedure. Laryngoscope 1974;84(4):568–77.
34. Jufas N, Treble A, Newey A, et al. Endoscopically guided transtympanic balloon catheter dilatation of the eustachian tube: a cadaveric pilot study. Otol Neurotol 2016;37(4):350–5.
35. Kepchar J, Acevedo J, Schroeder J, et al. Transtympanic balloon dilatation of eustachian tube: a human cadaver pilot study. J Laryngol Otol 2012;126(11):1102–7.
36. Oh S-J, Lee I-W, Goh E-K, et al. Trans-tympanic catheter insertion for treatment of patulous eustachian tube. Am J Otolaryngol 2015;36(6):748–52.

Eustachian Tube Function

Bernard Ars, MD, PhD[a], Joris Dirckx, PhD[b,*]

KEYWORDS

- Physiology of the eustachian tube
- Balance of pressure variations in the middle ear cleft
- Fibrocartilaginous eustachian tube
- Morphofunctional partition of the middle ear cleft

KEY POINTS

- The fibrocartilaginous eustachian tube is part of a system of contiguous organs including the nose, palate, rhinopharynx, and middle ear cleft.
- It is not a simple tube, but a complex organ consisting of a dynamic conduit with its mucosa, cartilage, surrounding soft tissue, peritubal muscles, and superior bony support (the sphenoid sulcus).
- The authors believe that the principal roles of the fibrocartilaginous eustachian tube could be the optimization of middle ear sound transmission and protection of the inner ear structures.

GENERAL INTRODUCTION

The fibrocartilaginous eustachian tube is part of a system of contiguous organs including the nose, palate, rhinopharynx, and middle ear cleft. The middle ear cleft consists of the tympanic cavity, which includes the bony eustachian tube (protympanum) and the mastoid gas cells system (**Fig. 1**). The tympanic cavity and mastoid gas cells are interconnected and allow gaseous exchange and pressure regulation.

The fibrocartilaginous eustachian tube is not a simple tube, but a complex organ consisting of a dynamic conduit with its mucosa, cartilage, surrounding soft tissue, peritubal muscles (ie, tensor and levator veli palatine, salpingopharyngeus and tensor tympani), and superior bony support (the sphenoid sulcus).

The authors think that the principal roles of the fibrocartilaginous eustachian tube could be the optimization of middle ear sound transmission and protection of the inner ear structures. These roles are aided by maintenance of the indispensable balance of pressure variations within the middle ear cleft, relative to ambient pressures. Given that the fibrocartilaginous eustachian tube links the protected sterile environment of

[a] University of Namur, c/o Avenue du Polo 68, Namur, Belgium; [b] Laboratory of Biomedical Physics, University of Antwerp, Groenenborgerlaan 171, Antwerpen 2020, Belgium
* Corresponding author.
E-mail address: joris.dirckx@uantwerpen.be

Otolaryngol Clin N Am 49 (2016) 1121–1133
http://dx.doi.org/10.1016/j.otc.2016.05.003
oto.theclinics.com

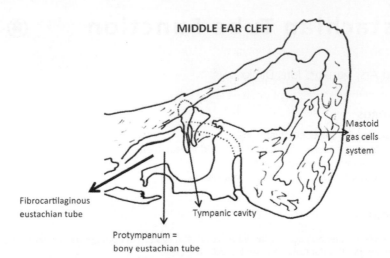

MIDDLE EAR CLEFT

Mastoid gas cells system

Fibrocartilaginous eustachian tube

Tympanic cavity

Protympanum = bony eustachian tube

Fig. 1. Section through the temporal bone: fibrocartilaginous eustachian tube and middle ear cleft: tympanic cavity with ossicles and mastoid gas cell system.

the middle ear cleft to the potentially hostile outside world, it must provide 3 additional specific organic functions, as follows:

- Mechanical protection against rhinopharyngeal secretions and pathogenic microorganism reflux, as well as against retrograde propagation of vocal sounds
- Local immune defense
- Mucociliary clearance into the rhinopharynx of secretions produced in the middle ear cleft and carried away in its inferior part.

Tubal function is an intrinsic and important component of the middle ear cleft pressure regulation system.

TUBAL MECHANICS

The proximal one-third of the tubal length is a bony funnel-shaped extension of the middle ear cleft, the protympanum, is narrowest at the isthmus.

The distal two-thirds of the tubal length is the pharyngeal portion, which is composed of a cartilaginous skeleton to which is attached a complex arrangement of peritubal muscles capable of a wide range of dynamic movements.

This cartilaginous portion is normally closed in the resting position because of apposition of the mucosal walls. Closure occurs over a variable length (5–10 mm) just a few millimeters distal to the bony isthmus where the cartilaginous skeleton becomes flexible.

This portion that intermittently dilates to the open position is termed the functional valve because this describes its purpose.[1]

Contraction of the levator veli palatine muscle raises the soft palate and medially rotates the medial cartilaginous lamina.[2,3] Contraction of the tensor veli palatine muscle tenses the anterolateral membranous wall and distracts it laterally to dilate the tubal valve into the open position.[4]

Intermittent brief tubal dilation is most likely the principal mechanism for equilibration of middle ear cleft pressure with the ambient atmosphere. Involuntary dilation of the fibrocartilaginous eustachian tube occurs throughout the day, typically occurring with a swallow or yawn, but it does not accompany every swallow or yawn. Barometric and chemical receptors within the middle ear cleft are thought to provide autonomic nervous system feedback that influences the frequency of involuntary tubal opening.[5,6]

Tubal dilation occurs in normal subjects approximately 1.4 times per minute during daytime, with the duration of opening averaging 0.4 seconds.[7] During sleep, the frequency of tubal opening is substantially reduced.

Sequential muscular contractions initiate rotational movements of the cartilaginous framework and create tension within the anterolateral wall, which causes the effacement of its resting bulge. This effacement is the primary action that opens the lumen to the middle ear cleft.[8]

Tubal dilation begins with the action of the levator veli palatine muscle to medially rotate the cartilaginous skeleton, primarily its mobile distal half of the medial cartilaginous lamina.[9] Tensor veli palatine muscle contraction follows, causing the resting convexity of the anterolateral wall to become effaced or even concave as the final step to transiently open the lumen.[10-12]

It is thought that intermittent brief dilation of the tube is the principal mechanism for equilibration of middle ear cleft pressure with the ambient atmosphere.[13-15] Middle ear cleft gas exchange is an ongoing process that continually generates a net absorption of gases resulting in an increasingly negative pressure between tubal dilations.[16-19] There is a gradient of partial pressures of gases between the middle ear cleft gases and the venous capillary soluble gases that drives the net absorption of gas into the circulation over time.

CO_2 has the highest coefficient of diffusion and is most rapidly exchanged with the net exchange passing from the venous blood to the middle ear cleft. The next most rapid diffusion occurs with O_2, passing from the middle ear cleft into the blood. Diffusing much more slowly into the circulation is N_2, the predominant partial pressure in both air and blood and the source of the largest gradient. It is the slow absorption of N_2 that causes the increasing relative vacuum between ambient air and the middle ear cleft over time.[20,21]

Intermittent dilation with opening of the middle ear cleft may principally serve to regulate nitrogen balance.[18]

Tubal dilation is likely naturally facilitated by the presence of surface tension–reducing substances that are found in its mucus. Surfactants are produced within the tubal mucosa and probably aid in reducing the surface tension of the lumen, which reduces the work required to dilate the tube.[22]

Fluid and secretions in the middle ear cleft are cleared by a combination of the muscular pumping action that occurs with the tubal closing process[23] and by mucociliary activity.[24] Reflux of rhinopharyngeal secretions into the middle ear cleft is limited or prevented by the closed position of the resting pharyngeal fibrocartilaginous eustachian tube and by the trapped volume of gas in the tympanic cavity and mastoid gas cells system, which creates a gas cushion. Reflux of the sounds of breathing and vocalization are similarly blocked by the closed resting position of the pharyngeal eustachian tube.

THE PLACE OF TUBAL PHYSIOLOGY IN PRESSURE BALANCING OF THE MIDDLE EAR CLEFT MORPHOFUNCTIONAL PARTITION

From the quantitative point of view, gas spaces of the middle ear cleft constitutes most of the pneumatic spaces of the temporal bone. The middle ear cleft consists of both the mastoid gas cells system and the tympanic cavity (see **Fig. 1**). The latter comprises the tympanum and 4 annexes: the epitympanum, hypotympanum, retrotympanum, and protympanum, which correspond with the bony eustachian tube. The middle ear cleft consists of a set of interconnected gas cells lined with the same respiratory mucosa. Because the gas exchange is performed through the mucosa of the cells, the total surface area of mucosa influences the rate of gas exchange.[25]

The tympanic cavity is constricted in its superior third by the interatticotympanic diaphragm, which is a bony membranous barrier perforated by 2 small permanent openings: the anterior tympanic isthmus, which is situated between the tensor tympani tendon and the stapes; and the posterior tympanic isthmus, which is between the double posterior ligament of the incus and the bony posterior tympanic wall.

This anatomic barrier divides the middle ear cleft into 2 separate compartments: an anteroinferior compartment, principally devoted to the mucociliary clearance function, and a posterosuperior compartments, more devoted to the gas exchange function. The barrier forms a diaphragm that is composed of 2 complementary types of structure: mucosal folds and bones with muscular and ligament structures, namely the head and neck of the malleus, the body and short process of the incus, the tensor tympani muscle, the anterior and lateral mallear, and the double posterior incudal ligaments (**Fig. 2**). This concept of partition makes it easier to understand the mechanisms involved in the pathogenesis of otitis media.[26,27] Clinical as well as surgical management is thereby enhanced.

The anteroinferior compartment of the middle ear cleft, which is situated under the diaphragm, includes the protympanum, mesotympanum, and hypotympanum, and is covered by secretory or nonsecretory ciliated cells that enable mucociliary clearance. It consists of a less rigid chamber because of the presence of the eardrum. Because of the fibrocartilaginous eustachian tube, it opens into an intermittently ventilated gas pocket. It communicates with the posterosuperior compartment by both the anterior and posterior tympanic isthmi. It is often the site of secondary bacterial infections from the rhinopharynx. An inflammatory process involving the mucosa of the anteroinferior middle ear cleft compartment leads to dysfunction in mucociliary clearance and to the accumulation of mucus (**Fig. 3**).

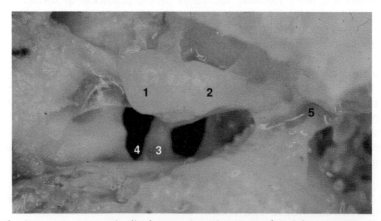

Fig. 2. The interatticotympanic diaphragm. Superior view of a right tympanic cavity in a fresh human temporal bone specimen. The tegmen tympani has been removed. (1) Malleus head, (2) body of the incus, (3) stapes, (4) anterior tympanic isthmus, (5) posterior tympanic isthmus.

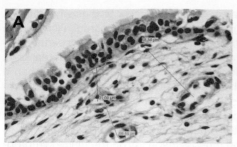 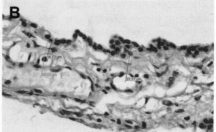

Fig. 3. Epithelium of the mucosa of the middle ear cleft. The 2 types of epithelium vary by site. (A) The anteroinferior compartment of the middle ear cleft has a pseudostratified epithelial layer with numerous mucous and ciliated cells. The connective tissue is thick and dense. (B) The posterosuperior compartment has a monocellular epithelial layer composed of only flat cells; there are no ciliated or mucous cells. The connective tissue is loose.

The posterosuperior compartment of the middle ear cleft, which is situated above the diaphragm, includes the epitympanum and retrotympanum, aditus ad antrum, antrum, and mastoid gas cells system. It is covered by a richly vascularized cuboidal epithelium that is devoted primarily to gas exchange. It consists of a rigid chamber and an open nonventilated gas pocket that communicates with the anteroinferior compartment via both openings. It may be the site of viral hematogenous infections. Inflammation of the mucosa of the posterosuperior middle ear cleft compartment impairs the gas exchange, which in turn leads to the development of a gas deficit in the middle ear cleft (compare with the peripheral and central nervous regulating system, as discussed later). The interatticotympanic diaphragm conditions the topography of the tympanic membrane retraction pockets. When only 1 opening is blocked, the posterosuperior quadrant of the pars tensa is attracted in the direction of the retrotympanum. When both openings are completely blocked, the pars flaccida is drawn in toward the epitympanum. In the same way, the diaphragm also influences the invasion of the middle ear cleft by a cholesteatoma.[16–21]

What, then, is the role of the mastoid? The physiology of the mastoid can only be understood in the context of balancing pressure variations in the middle ear cleft. The middle ear cleft is essentially a noncollapsible, poorly ventilated gas pocket through which sound wave energy is transported to reach the inner ear. All gases must be contained in a three-dimensional container or volume (V). The pressure (P) of a gas is created by the molecules of gas striking the walls of the container. It is a force per unit of area. The physical characteristics of a gas are linked by the ideal gas law: $PV = nRT$, in which n is the amount of gas expressed in moles, R is the universal gas constant, and T is the absolute temperature. The middle ear cleft is submitted to physiologic variations in volume and pressure. It has the capacity to maintain a steady state in volume and pressure, which is achieved by various regulatory mechanisms that neutralize or minimize the pressure and volume variations by adjusting the quantity of gas, its diffusion, and/or the volume of the middle ear cleft.[28]

Gas Exchanges

The gas content of the middle ear cleft is constituted and maintained by gas exchanges between the middle ear cleft and the neighboring structures, including the environment across the tympanic membrane, the inner ear via the round window membrane, the blood compartment via the mucosa, and the rhinopharynx through the fibrocartilaginous eustachian tube.[15,29–35]

The gases that are present in the middle ear cleft are identical to those found in the blood and in the atmosphere: oxygen (O_2), carbon dioxide (CO_2), nitrogen (N_2), argon (Ar), and water vapor (H_2O). Their relative amounts may be expressed by their partial pressure P(x). Nitrogen is neither produced nor consumed at the level of the middle ear cleft. The P(O_2) in the middle ear cleft is slightly lower and the P(CO_2) is slightly higher than in venous blood. This difference means that there is a modest consumption of O_2 and production of CO_2 in the middle ear cleft. Oxygen and nitrogen are absorbed from the middle ear cleft via the mucosa into the blood compartment. Carbon dioxide and water vapor are diffused from the blood compartment, via the mucosa, into the middle ear cleft.

The steady exchange of gas through the mucosa depends on the functional properties of the cells of the mucosa; the specific diffusion rate of the gas, which is a constant value for a particular gas; and the behavior of the vascular system. The primary purpose of the mucosa is to facilitate gas exchange between the middle ear cleft and the blood compartment through a constitutive tissular barrier.

To vibrate in an optimal manner, the tympano-ossicular system must remain in balance, which means that the intra–middle ear cleft pressure must be equivalent to the atmospheric pressure (760 mm Hg). In ambient air, this equivalent value is obtained by calculating the sum of the partial pressures of the 4 main constitutive gases in the air: oxygen (158 mm Hg), carbon dioxide (0.3 mm Hg), nitrogen (596 mm Hg), and water vapor (5.7 mm Hg).[36]

However, in the middle ear cleft, the composition of gas varies for 2 main reasons. The middle ear cleft is a closed cavity that is connected with the nasal cavities by the fibrocartilaginous eustachian tube. The gas in the rhinopharynx, which enters the middle ear cleft via the tube, consists of exhaled gas that contains less oxygen and more carbon dioxide than ambient air. This gas composition also varies because gas diffusion occurs between the middle ear cleft and the arterial and venous blood, via the mucosa. In blood, the partial pressures of these gases differ. There is more oxygen in the arterial blood (93 mm Hg) and more carbon dioxide in the venous blood (44 mm Hg) because the gas exchange occurs at the level of the pulmonary air cells and the tissues throughout the body, respectively.

Thus, the composition of gas in the middle ear cleft differs from that in ambient air. The gradient out from middle ear cleft to the capillaries is 57 mm Hg for oxygen, and the gradient in from the capillaries to the middle ear cleft is 39 mm Hg for carbon dioxide. These gradients should result in a negative pressure in the middle ear cleft. However, in spite of the difference in gas composition, the pressure in the middle ear cleft approximates the atmospheric pressure to enable optimal sound transmission.

The reason for this balance is 3-fold:

- Because the sum of the partial pressures of oxygen and carbon dioxide is lower in the middle ear cleft (90 mm Hg) than in ambient air (150 mm Hg), nitrogen exerts the higher partial pressure in the middle ear cleft (623 mm Hg) because of its slow diffusion toward the capillaries.
- The composition of the exhaled gas that enters the middle ear cleft via the tube contains less oxygen and more carbon dioxide than ambient air, and this reduces the passive diffusion of these gases through the mucosa.
- The blood flow through the middle ear cleft mucosa is probably low, which limits the importance of gas diffusion and enables the oxygen and carbon dioxide partial pressures to nearly equalize, because each has a high diffusion rate. The same mechanism applies to water vapor, for which the diffusion rate is also very high. Transmucosal gas exchange results in gas absorption.

Regulating Systems

The steady state in volume and pressure into the middle ear cleft is preserved by 2 types of regulating mechanisms: the in situ adaptation systems, and both central and peripheral nervous regulating systems with retrocontrol between the middle ear cleft and the muscles of the fibrocartilaginous eustachian tube.

The in situ adaptation systems

The in situ adaptation systems consist mainly of the compliance of the tympanic membrane lamina propria, the fibrocartilaginous eustachian tube function, and the behavior of the vascular system of the middle ear cleft mucosa, especially that of the mastoid.

The compliance of the tympanic membrane lamina propria The compliance of the tympanic membrane lamina propria is used in sudden pressure changes (eg, altitude, flight, diving, explosions) This compliance occurs largely because of the viscoelastic properties of the lamina propria and the flexibility of the incudomalleolar joint, which acts as a static pressure receptor for the tympanic membrane, ensuring three-dimensional movement into the malleus. Deformation of the eardrum causes a volume change of the semirigid middle ear cleft and can therefore compensate partially for fast pressure changes. The eardrum is an active pressure buffer but also a passive pressure victim.[37–41]

The fibrocartilaginous eustachian tube function The fibrocartilaginous eustachian tube is closed most of the time, and it therefore does not function as a ventilation hole, which keeps pressure inside the middle ear cleft equal to the outside. Only at large pressure differences, more than 2 kPa, does the fibrocartilaginous eustachian tube open spontaneously.

Changes in position seem to affect the function of the fibrocartilaginous eustachian tube. The mean volume of gas passing through the tube in the upright position is reduced by one-third when the body is elevated at 20° to the horizontal position. It is reduced by two-thirds in the horizontal position. This difference is the result of the increase in the venous tissular pressure around the fibrocartilaginous eustachian tube.[42]

The vascular system in combination with the mastoid gas cell system The behavior of the vascular system plays an important regulatory role in the physiologic balance of pressure variations in the middle ear cleft. Variations in the middle ear cleft blood flow, associated with variations in the permeability of the vessels, allow ample adaptation to normal gas pressure fluctuations.[43,44] The normal extensive variations regularly observed in middle ear cleft pressure over a 24-hour period are related to the vascular adaptations required by body position and sleep. The mastoid gas cell system constitutes the most important volume of the middle ear cleft and therefore represents the major part of the middle ear cleft mucosal area available for vascular gas exchange.[45]

The amount of gas present in the mastoid is important in regulating middle ear cleft pressure for 2 reasons. First, the physical, anatomic, properties of mastoid volume affect compliance: the greater the volume, the more compliant the system. Second, the surface area affects mucosal gas exchanges. Both are important in the regulation of middle ear cleft pressure. The gas contained in the mastoid gas cells system acts as a physiologic passive pressure buffer.

The size of the mastoid gas cells system varies greatly between individuals. However, whatever the cause, be it genetic determination of growth or environmental factors, there is unanimous agreement that the small mastoid gas cell system has a pathologic association. The smaller the system, the faster the deviation from normal pressures. However, nature is a matter of balance. It is not a question of determining the volume of the mastoid in order to predict its clinical potential. In normal conditions and with healthy mucosa, a small mastoid in an adult is normal in that it constitutes the complete outcome of normal and standard development (ie, the individual simply possesses the morphologic characteristic of being small). A small mastoid in an adult is normal, in that it is sufficient for the physiologic balance of pressure variations in the middle ear cleft. This small mastoid is no more likely to develop disorder than another is. However, when the mucosa undergoes an inflammatory process, a small mastoid in an adult (eg, as an outcome of disturbed or failed development) is at a disadvantage when it is exposed to excessive variations in pressure. This mastoid is too small compared with the rest of the middle ear cleft. Fluctuations in middle ear cleft pressure in the presence of a small mastoid gas cells system result in greater forces applied to the tympanic membrane, compared with the same pressure changes in a larger mastoid gas cells system. If the expansion reservoir is too small, it cannot play its role adequately.

In normal conditions and healthy mucosa, a slight negative pressure is present in the middle ear cleft compared with the outside air, created by exchanges of gas between the cleft and the blood compartment. Gas exchanges through the mucosa of the middle ear cleft are induced by the gradient of partial pressure of gases between the cleft and the capillaries of the submucosal connective tissue. Given the capacity of gas diffusion in the middle ear cleft, partial pressures of those gases establish a balance on both sides of the mucosal barrier of the middle ear cleft. The progressive diffusion of the gases is capable of modifying the gas composition in the middle ear cleft as well as in the circulating blood. The gas that penetrates into the middle ear cleft from the rhinopharynx is not outside air. Its composition is close to exhaled air. Quantitatively, the main gas that enters the middle ear cleft is nitrogen. Nitrogen diffuses much more slowly in the blood than the other gases (35 times more slowly than CO_2 and 1.8 times more slowly than O_2)[46,47] **(Fig. 4)**.

Considering this nitrogen in steady state, there is a difference in partial pressure between the middle ear cleft and the blood flow around the middle ear cleft. This steady state corresponds more or less with the total pressure difference (54–56 mm Hg) between the middle ear cleft and blood. In steady state, oxygen, carbon dioxide, and

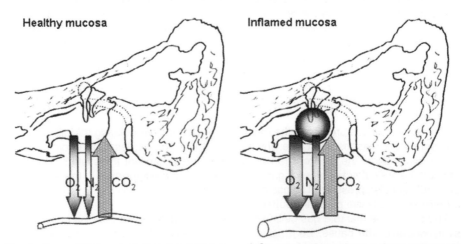

Fig. 4. Gas exchanges between the middle ear cleft and the blood compartment through healthy and inflamed mucosa.

water vapor have nearly the same partial pressures in the middle ear cleft as in the blood compartment. Consequently, an increase in blood flow into the middle ear cleft has little effect on exchanges of these gases, except perhaps during the night, when carbon dioxide level increases and oxygen becomes reduced in blood flow. In contrast, nitrogen always maintains a higher partial pressure into the middle ear cleft compared with the blood. Therefore, there is a clear and continuous elimination of nitrogen from the middle ear cleft in the direction of the blood compartment. This elimination leads to the negative pressure bias in the middle ear cleft. In normal conditions, this elimination is regularly compensated for by the gas contribution originating from the rhinopharynx. A variation in blood flow could consequently explain variations in nitrogen absorption.

The peripheral and central nervous regulating systems
In the middle ear cleft, the steady state in volume and pressure close to the atmospheric pressure is maintained not only by the in situ adaptation systems but also by a peripheral and central nervous regulating system with retrocontrol between the middle ear cleft and the muscles of the fibrocartilaginous eustachian tube.

The mucosa of the middle ear cleft manages the quality of the gas contained in the middle ear cleft, especially its composition, mainly by means of chemosensitive sensors that act on the neurocapillary system.

The fibrocartilaginous eustachian tube manages the quantity (volume) of the gas contained in the middle ear cleft by means of barosensitive sensors that act on the neuromuscular system.

Sensors located in the middle ear cleft
Chemosensors Within the middle ear cleft, the innervation of the mucosa originates from the autonomic nervous system, which gives and receives information at the same time from sympathetic and parasympathetic networks.[48,49]

Adrenergic nerve endings have been identified, most of them in the vicinity of vessels. They probably control their tonus. The peptidergic system, nonadrenergic and noncholinergic, also plays a role. The presence of peptidergic mediators such as substance P, vasoactive intestinal peptide, or calcitonin gene–related peptide has been shown. It has been established that these mediators give rise to vasodilatation as well as an increase in the vascular permeability.

At the level of the middle ear cleft, chemosensors situated within the glomic tissue of the mucosa explain variations in the gas composition and contribute to gas transfer from the rhinopharynx in the direction of the middle ear cleft.

Barosensors The presence of barosensors has been reported at the level of the middle ear cleft as well as at the level of the tympanic membrane.

At the level of the tympanic membrane, stretch-sensitive sensors have been described. These sensors are corpuscles situated in the lamina propria. Their sensitivity should fit the tympanic membrane movements. Moreover, they might play a role in the detection of pressure variations in the middle ear cleft.[6,50–54]

The tensor tympani muscle does not seem to be involved in active dilatation of the fibrocartilaginous eustachian tube. However, there may be stretch sensors in the tympanic membrane that could be related to modulation of the middle ear cleft pressure through the tensor tympani muscle, thereby affecting the tensor veli palatine muscle opening of the fibrocartilaginous eustachian tube.[55]

Sensors located at the pharyngeal orifice of the fibrocartilaginous eustachian tube Opening of the fibrocartilaginous eustachian tube occurs when there is pressure imbalance on both sides of the tympanic membrane.[56]

Barosensors are situated in the vicinity of the pharyngeal orifice of the fibrocartilaginous eustachian tube,[57] and also within the middle ear cleft and most likely in the tympanic membrane. In this way, there may be a neural connection between the sensory sensors in the tympanic membrane and the tubal muscles.

The opening of the fibrocartilaginous eustachian tube may not be limited to a movement associated with or connected to yawning or swallowing, but could be controlled by a system whose retrocontrol could be initiated in the tympanic membrane.

Neural connection between sensors The presence of a feedback system has been described, acting from the middle ear cleft to the tubal muscles as well as afferent nerves from the sensors located in the middle ear cleft to the salivary nucleus of the brain stem. This nucleus also receives the efferent fibers of both the sensitive and sensorial sensibilities from nerves V and IX. This nucleus also provides efferent fibers to the swallowing muscles as well as fibers that regulate the vasomotor tonus of the arteriole and precapillary sphincters from the active tissular areas (mainly the mastoidian areas). Therefore, this system is consistent with the description of a complex system with a regulation loop with central nervous control.[5,58–60]

How the System Operates

The gas exchange that governs the balance of middle ear cleft pressure variations is performed mainly in the mucosa of the middle ear cleft and through the fibrocartilaginous eustachian tube.

In the middle ear cleft, the steady state in volume and pressure is maintained close to atmospheric pressure, by the working of local mechanisms of adaptability and also by regulation from both central and peripheral nervous systems with retrocontrol between the middle ear cleft and the muscles of the fibrocartilaginous eustachian tube.

The middle ear cleft is a poorly ventilated but highly perfused organ. Gas exchanges depend on variations in middle ear cleft blood flow. In a similar fashion to alveoli in the

---

Box 1
Conclusions

- The fibrocartilaginous eustachian tube has a valvelike function, with the mucosal surfaces in apposition in the resting position.

- The tubal muscles must actively dilate the tubal valve open in order for adequate gas exchanges into the middle ear cleft to occur.

- At first, in normal conditions, the healthy mucosa of the middle ear cleft provides an intermittent supply of gas, by a regular, periodic, active process of gas transfer into the middle ear cleft.

- Gas transfer via the tube is poor, compared with the delicate and perfectly controlled gas exchanges between the middle ear cleft and blood compartment, via the mucosa.

- A second situation occurs for healthy mucosa of the middle ear cleft in exceptional situations, such as when at altitude, flying, or diving, or in accidental situations such as explosions. In these situations, the tube plays the leading role in balancing the variations of pressure in the middle ear cleft. It is a highly sophisticated security valve.
  It serves as a release valve for excessive positive pressure in the middle ear cleft, and, by means of muscular forces, opens to equalize excessive negative pressure in the middle ear

- A third condition occurs when the mucosa undergoes an inflammatory process. With regard to the gas supply to the middle ear cleft, the main process occurs at the level of the middle ear cleft mucosa.

lung, the direction of gas exchange is predicated on the differences in partial pressure of the component gases in the middle ear cleft and in the blood compartment.

When the mucosa is healthy, there is a balance of gas exchanges because oxygen and nitrogen are absorbed by the mucosa at the same rate at which carbon dioxide is expelled. For a given mucosal blood flow, nitrogen is the exchange rate–limiting factor for middle ear gas loss, because it diffuses slower than carbon dioxide and oxygen, which equilibrate quickly with venous blood (**Box 1**).

REFERENCES

1. Poe D, Pyykko I, Valtonen H, et al. Analysis of Eustachian tube function by video endoscopy. Am J Otol 2000;21(5):602–7.
2. Rich A. A physiological study of the Eustachian tube and its related muscles. Bull 1920;31:3005–10.
3. Proctor B. Anatomy of the Eustachian tube. Arch Otolaryngol 1973;97(1):2–8.
4. Rood S, Doyle J. Morphology of tensor veli palatine, tensor tympani and dilatator tubae muscles. Ann Otol Rhinol Laryngol 1978;87:202–10.
5. Eden A, Gannon P. Neural control of middle ear aeration. Arch Otolaryngol Head Neck Surg 1987;113(2):133–7.
6. Rockley T, Hawke W. The middle ear as a baroreceptor. Acta Otolaryngol 1992;112(5):816–23.
7. Mondain M, Vidal D. Monitoring Eustachian tube opening: preliminary results in normal subjects. Laryngoscope 1997;107(10):1414–9.
8. Bluestone C, Bluestone M. Eustachian tube: structure, function, role in otitis media. Hamilton (Canada); Lewiston (NY): BC Decker; 2005. p. 113–50.
9. Cantekin E, Doyle W. Effect of levator veli palatine muscle excision on eustachian tube function. Acta Otolaryngol 1983;109(5):281–4.
10. Honjo I, Okazaki N. Experimental study of the Eustachian tube function with regard to its related muscles. Acta Otolaryngol 1979;87(1–2):84–9.
11. Honjo I, Ushiro K. Role of the tensor tympani muscle in Eustachian tube function. Acta Otolaryngol 1983;95(3–4):329–32.
12. Ghadiali S, Swarts J. Effect of tensor veli palatini muscles paralysis on Eustachian tube mechanics. Ann Otol Rhinol Laryngol 2003;112(8):704–11.
13. Sade J. Eustachian tube function. Acta Otolaryngol Suppl 1984;414:83–4.
14. Honjo I. Eustachian tube and middle ear diseases. Tokyo: Springer-Verlag; 1988.
15. Hergils L, Magnusson B. Nasal composition in humans and its implication on middle ear pressure. Acta Otolaryngol 1998;118(5):697–700.
16. Felding J, Rasmussen B. Gas composition of the normal and the ventilated middle ear cavity. Scand J Clin Lab Invest Suppl 1987;186:31–41.
17. Ostfeld E, Silverberg A. Gas composition and pressure in the middle ear: a model for the physiological steady state. Laryngoscope 1991;101(3):297–304.
18. Ars B, Ars-Piret N. Middle ear pressure balance under normal conditions. Specific role of the middle ear structures. Acta Otorhinolaryngol Belg 1994;48(4):339–42.
19. Doyle W, Seroky J. Middle ear gas exchange in rhesus monkeys. Ann Otol Rhinol Laryngol 1994;103(8):636–45.
20. Tideholm B. Middle ear cleft pressure. In: Ars B, editor. Fibrocartilaginous Eustachian tube – middle ear cleft. The Hague (Netherlands): Kugler Publications; 2003. p. 97–112.
21. Pau H, Sievert U. Pressure changes in the human middle ear without opening the Eustachian tube. Acta Otolaryngol 2009;129(11):1182–6.

22. Birken E, Brookler K. Surface tension lowering substance of the canine Eustachian tube. Ann Otol Rhinol Laryngol 1972;81(2):268–71.

23. Honjo I, Hayashi M. Pumping and clearance function of the Eustachian tube. Am J Otolaryngol 1985;6(3):241–4.

24. Bluestone C. Otitis media, atelectasis and Eustachian tube dysfunction. In: Bluestone CD, Stool SE, Kenna MA, editors. Pediatric otolaryngology. Philadelphia: WB Saunders; 1996. p. 389–90.

25. Ars B. Balance of pressure variation in the middle ear cleft. In: Ars B, editor. Fibrocartilaginous eustachian tube – middle ear cleft. Amsterdam: Kugler Publications; 2003. p. 57–66.

26. Ars B. Chronic otitis media. Pathogenesis-oriented therapeutic management. Amsterdam: Kugler Publications; 2008.

27. Ars B. Middle ear cleft: three structural sets, two functional sets. Otorhinolaryngol Nova 1998;8(6):273–6.

28. Piiper J. Physiological equilibria of gas cavities in the body. In: Fenn W, Rahn H, editors. Handbook of physiology, section 3: respiration. Washington, DC: American Physiological Society; 1965. p. 1205–18.

29. Elner A. Normal gas exchange in the human middle ear. Ann Otol Rhinol Laryngol 1976;85:161–4.

30. Hergils L, Magnuson B. Middle ear gas composition in pathologic conditions: mass spectrometry in otitis media with effusion and atelectasis. Ann Otol Rhinol Laryngol 1997;106:743–5.

31. Ingestedt S, Ivarsson A, Jonson B. Mechanics of the human middle ear. Pressure regulation in aviation and diving. A non-traumatic method. Acta Otolaryngol 1967; 228S:221–58.

32. Luntz M, Sadé J. Dynamic measurement of gas composition in the middle ear. I. Technique. Acta Otolaryngol 1993;113:349–52.

33. Sadé J, Ar A. Middle ear and auditory tube: middle ear clearance, gas exchange, and pressure regulation. Otolaryngol Head Neck Surg 1997;116:499–524.

34. Sadé J, Luntz M. Dynamic measurement of gas composition in the middle ear. Steady state values. Acta Otolaryngol 1993;113:353–7.

35. Tideholm B, Jönsson S, Carlborg B, et al. Continuous 24-hour measurement of middle ear pressure. Acta Otolaryngol 1996;116:581–8.

36. Doyle J. Middle ear pressure regulation. In: Rosowski J, Merchant S, editors. The function and mechanics of normal, diseased and reconstructed middle ears. The Hague (The Netherlands): Kugler Publications; 2000. p. 3–21.

37. Ars B, Decraemer W, Ars-Piret N. The lamina propria and cholesteatoma. Clin Otolaryngol 1989;14:471–5.

38. Ars B, Dirckx J, Decraemer W, et al. Faulty aeration of the middle ear cavities and subsequent behavior of the tympanic membrane. Conference on the Eustachian tube and middle ear diseases. Geneva, Switzerland, October 20–29, 1989; Amsterdam/Berkeley/Milano: Kugler & Ghedini Publications; 1989, p. 365–71.

39. Dirckx J, Decraemer W. Human tympanic membrane deformation under static pressure. Hear Res 1990;51:93–106.

40. Dirckx J, Decraemer W, Larsson CH, et al. Volume displacement of the Mongolian gerbil pars flaccida as a function of pressure. Hear Res 1998;118:35–46.

41. Sadé J. Hyperectasis: the hyperinflated tympanic membrane: the middle ear as an actively controlled system. Otol Neurotol 2001;22:133–9.

42. Miura M, Takahashi H, Sugimaru T, et al. Influence of surface condition of mucosa of Eustachian tube on tubal compliance. Acta Otolaryngol 1996;116:840–4.

43. Alper C, Tabari R, Seroky J, et al. Effects of dopamine, dobutamine and phentolamine on middle ear pressure and blood flow in cynomolgus monkeys. Acta Otolaryngol 1995;115:55–60.
44. Luntz M, Levi D, Sadé J, et al. Relationship between the gas composition of the middle ear and the venous blood at steady state. Laryngoscope 1995;105:510–2.
45. Dirckx JJJ, Gaihede M, Jacobsen H, et al. Pressure fluctuations in the normal and intact middle ear and its relation to speed of transmucosal gas exchange. In: Ars B, editor. Chronic otitis media. pathogenesis-oriented therapeutic management. Amsterdam: Kugler Publications; 2008. p. 155–70.
46. Doyle J. The mastoid as a functional rate-limiter of middle ear pressure change. Int J Pediatr Otorhinolaryngol 2007;71:393–402.
47. Kania R. Modélisation expérimentale et mathématique des échanges gazeux transmuqueux de l'oreille moyenne en conditions normales et inflammatoires. Thèse de Doctorat de l'Université de Paris 6; 2006. p. 1–155.
48. Ar A, Herman PH, Lecain E, et al. Middle ear gas loss in inflammatory conditions: the role of mucosa thickness and blood flow. Respir Physiolo Neurobiol 2007;155: 167–76.
49. Ito J, Oyagi S, Honso I. Autonomic innervations in the middle ear and pharynx. Acta Otolaryngol 1993;506S:90–3.
50. Widemar L, Hellstrom S, Schultzberg M, et al. Autonomic innervation of the tympanic membrane. An immunocytochemical and histofluorescence study. Acta Otolaryngol 1985;100:58–65.
51. Lim D, Jackson D, Bennett J. Human middle ear corpuscles. A light and electron microscopic study. Laryngoscope 1975;85:1725–37.
52. Nagai T. Innervation of the tympanic membrane. Acta Otorhinolaryngol Belg 1995;49:117–20.
53. Nagai T, Tono T. Encapsulated nerve corpuscles in the human tympanic membrane. Arch Otorhinolaryngol 1989;246:169–72.
54. Wilson J. The nerves and nerve endings in the membrane tympani. J Comp Neurol 1907;17:459–68.
55. Gannon P, Eden A. A specialized innervation of the tensor tympani muscle in *Macaca fascicularis*. Brain Res 1987;404:257–62.
56. Poe D. Opening and closure of the fibrocartilaginous eustachian tube. In: Ars B, editor. Fibrocartilaginous eustachian tube – middle ear cleft. The Hague (The Netherlands): Kugler Publications; 2003. p. 49–56.
57. Gumidi G. Nasopharyngeal mecano-receptors and their role in autoregulation of endolymphatic pressure. ORL 1981;60:43–56.
58. Eden A, Laitman J, Gannon P. Mechanisms of middle ear aeration: anatomic and physiologic evidence in primates. Laryngoscope 1990;100:67–75.
59. Estève D. Tubomanometry and pathology. In: Ars B, editor. Fibrocartilaginous Eustachian tube – middle ear cleft. The Hague (The Netherlands): Kugler Publications; 2003. p. 159–75.
60. Gaihede M. Determination of middle ear pressure in diseased ears. In: Dirckx J, Sadé J. Middle ear pressure regulation: basic research and clinical observation. Otol Neurotol 2005;26:300–9.

Preoperative and Intraoperative Evaluation of the Eustachian Tube in Chronic Ear Surgery

Muaaz Tarabichi, MD*, Mustafa Kapadia, MD

KEYWORDS

- Eustachian tube obstruction • Cholesteatoma • Tympanic perforation
- Tympanoplasty • CT of temporal bone • Valsalva maneuver

KEY POINTS

- Mechanical obstruction of the eustachian tube is a common finding in chronic ear surgery and needs to be assessed preoperatively for the purpose of informed consent and for making a plan of action.
- Valsalva computed tomography of the temporal bone is helpful in assessing the patency of the distal end of the eustachian tube.
- Intraoperative inspection of the protympanic segment of the eustachian tube is possible and might lead to clear determination of the site of obstruction.
- Measurement of the opening pressure of the eustachian tube is a useful determinant of the presence of obstruction and the effect of possible interventions.

 Video content accompanies this article at http://www.oto.theclinics.com.

INTRODUCTION

Surgery for chronic ear disease has always centered on disease removal and restoration of hearing without paying much attention to the underlying eustachian tube disorder. Because much of the eustachian tube is out of reach of traditional instruments, it is always assumed that time and age have resolved the disorder.[1] Failures in surgery for chronic ear disease have been shown to correlate with persistent eustachian tube dysfunction.[2] So far, there is no reliable, reproducible, and simple way of assessing the function of the eustachian tube.[3] The anatomic patency of the tube can be assessed by testing for opening pressure[4] and further localization of possible obstruction obtained by Valsalva computed tomography (CT) and endoscopic evaluation of

ENT Clinic, American Hospital Dubai, PO Box 5566, Oud Mehta Road, Dubai, United Arab Emirates
* Corresponding author.
E-mail address: mtarabichi@ahdubai.com

Otolaryngol Clin N Am 49 (2016) 1135–1147
http://dx.doi.org/10.1016/j.otc.2016.05.004
0030-6665/16/$ – see front matter © 2016 Elsevier Inc. All rights reserved.
oto.theclinics.com

protympanum.[5] Endoscopic technique and its excellent access to the tympanic cavity allows the identification and assessment of other sites of segmental failure of ventilation within the temporal bone.[6] This article discusses the authors' algorithm for both preoperative and intraoperative evaluation of patency of the eustachian tube and assessment of any segmental ventilation failures in patients with chronic ear disorders.

Valsalva Computed Tomography

Many of the testing methods that have been devised for eustachian tube function are not anatomically based and are indirect methods that do not locate the site of obstruction.[3] Indirect evidence of the tube status on CT is usually derived from the status and pneumatization of the middle ear cleft. There has been some success at MRI visualization of eustachian tube structure and related muscles, as well as the depiction of submucosal tumors, but the lumen and physical obstruction could not be visualized in the naturally collapsed tube.[7]

In normal physiologic conditions, the eustachian tube opens as a result of a combination of direct muscle action and indirect action by increased nasopharyngeal pressure beyond the opening pressure of the tube.[8] Improved CT technology with spiral CT has resulted in a very short imaging time that allows patients to maintain Valsalva maneuver throughout the examination.[9] In addition, multiplanar reconstruction allows orientation of the plane in the desired way to match the sloping position of the eustachian tube. Valsalva CT of the temporal bone is performed while the patient is actively performing the Valsalva maneuver (concurrent with the examination). Upright positioning of the patient (as is possible in cone beam CT) enhances the patient's ability to dilate the tube. Technologists are instructed to ask the patient to perform forceful exhalation against a closed nose. Primary image acquisition is made with the patient in the supine position using helical mode and a 0.6 mm (thickness) by 0.5 mm (increment) overlapping axial data set is usually obtained. Multiplanar reconstruction of the images in the axis of the eustachian tube is then performed. Different makers have proprietary software on the CT scanner workstation that use the following methodology: the rotation center (crosshair) is positioned at the fundus of the nasopharyngeal end of the eustachian tube on axial sections. Then, looking at the sagittal view, the axial plane is tilted anteroinferiorly until the whole length of the tube is visualized (**Fig. 1**). Visualization of the whole length of the cartilaginous tube with Valsalva is usually observed in almost a third of the normal population. This phenomenon tends to be bilateral in patients who have it. In almost all patients, Valsalva maneuver increases the length of the visualized segment and extends it to include the distal one-third of the tube. Therefore, a collapsed distal tube despite adequate performance of Valsalva maneuver during CT indicates distal eustachian tube obstruction. In clinical practice, this is consistently observed in association with enlarged adenoids filling the fossa of Rosenmüller and collapsing the torus tubarius anteriorly (**Fig. 2**). This finding represents an unusual cause of eustachian tube obstruction in patients with chronic otitis media.

- Valsalva CT distends and visualizes the full length of the eustachian tube in one-third of the normal population; it is usually bilateral in patients who have it. The distal one-third of the tube is open on Valsalva CT in most normal patients.

Case discussion

This adult male patient presented to our clinic for left-sided middle ear effusion and retraction with a previous history of left ear blockage throughout his life and no nasal symptoms. His Valsalva CT confirmed the collapse of the distal eustachian tube

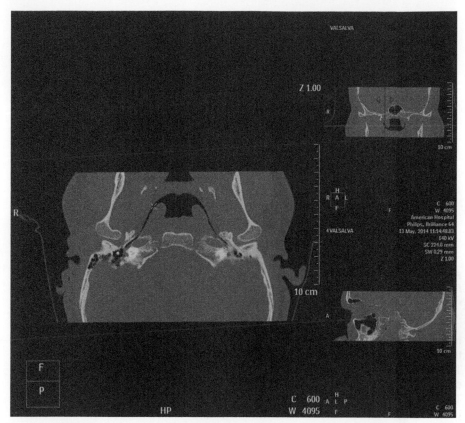

Fig. 1. Screenshot of CT workstation with full visualization of the whole length of the tube on multiplanar reconstruction. Multiplanar reconstruction of the images in the axis of the tube: the cross denoting the rotation center was positioned at the fundus of the nasopharyngeal end of the tube on axial sections. Then, looking at the sagittal view, the axial plane was tilted anteroinferiorly until the whole length of the tube was visualized.

secondary to enlarged adenoids that obliterated the fossa of Rosenmüller on the left side (see **Fig. 2**). Placement of tympanostomy tubes in the left ear was done in the clinic and middle ear effusion was evacuated. Using an endotracheal tube pressure pump, the pressure in the ear canal and the middle ear (through the tympanostomy tube) were increased to 50 cm H_2O while performing CT scan. **Fig. 3** shows the tube and the pressure pump in the axial plane. **Fig. 4** shows an anteroinferiorly angled view matching the position of the eustachian tube. Visualization of the protympanic segment of the eustachian tube and the isthmus area with air was obtained, showing patency of the proximal eustachian tube. The patient underwent microscopic adenoidectomy and decompression of the fossa of Rosenmüller, as seen in Video 1. Follow-up after 1 year shows the extrusion of tympanostomy tube, the healing of the tympanic membrane and the resolution of middle ear effusion.

COMPUTED TOMOGRAPHY ASSESSMENT OF SEGMENTAL VENTILATION FAILURES

Although eustachian tube dysfunction might be the initiating event, other sites of obstruction exist within the ventilation pathways of the middle ear cleft and can be a cause of segmental disease even in the presence of normal eustachian tube

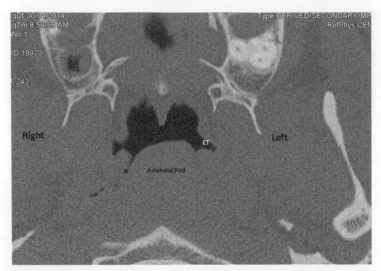

Fig. 2. Axial CT of the temporal bone showing the large adenoids and the filling of the left fossa of Rosenmüller despite the Valsalva technique. ET, nasopharyngeal opening of the eustachian tube; R, fossa of Rosenmüller on the right side.

function. **Fig. 5** shows a three-dimensional reconstruction of air-containing spaces of the temporal bone in a patient performing Valsalva and dilating his eustachian tube. The most upstream source of ventilation failure of the air cell system is the distal eustachian tube and the most downstream part of the system is the mastoid air cell system. The narrowest segment of the ventilation system is located in 2 places or isthmuses: the isthmus of the eustachian tube, and the tympanic isthmus. Both occur within, and in close proximity to, any recurrent childhood inflammatory and infectious middle ear disease with ample opportunity for scarring and inflammatory narrowing and closure. The tympanic isthmus is the space between the incudostapedial joint and the tensor

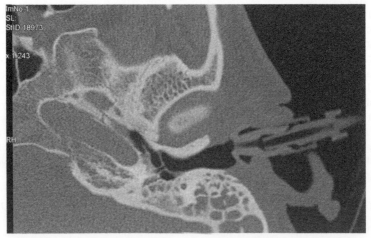

Fig. 3. Axial section of the left ear showing the tympanostomy tube and the pressure pump sealing the ear canal.

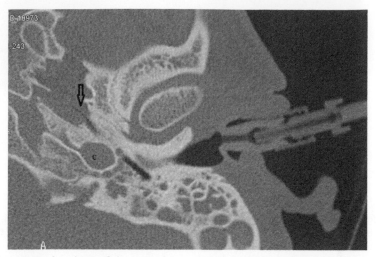

Fig. 4. Section in the plane of the eustachian tube of the left ear showing air in the area of the isthmus (*arrow*). C, carotid artery.

tympani tendon (**Fig. 6**). It is the channel for ventilation of the attic and mastoid cavity proper (**Fig. 7**). In most patients and anatomic specimens, all other routes of ventilation between the mastoid and the tympanic cavity are sealed by the epitympanic diaphragm. The diaphragm consists of the lateral incudomallear fold and lateral mallear fold closing off the lateral attic and therefore isolating it from the mesotympanum (**Fig. 8**). Anteriorly in the attic, the tensor fold is the second component of the epitympanic diaphragm and it blocks direct ventilation of the attic toward the eustachian tube

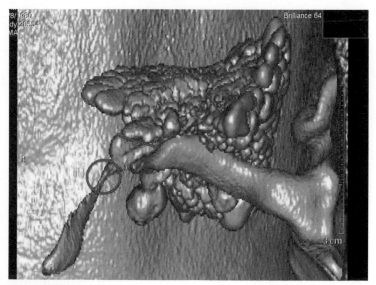

Fig. 5. Three-dimensional reconstruction of the air-containing spaces of the middle ear of a Valsalva CT scan. The red circle indicates the eustachian tube isthmus, and the red line indicates the tympanic isthmus.

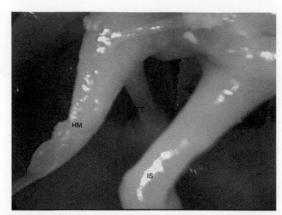

Fig. 6. Right ear: View through the isthmus with a 30° endoscope. CO, the COG; HM, handle of malleus; IS, incudostapedial joint; RE, the recess formed through the insertion of the fold anterior to the COG; TF, tensor fold; TT, tendon of the tensor tympani.

(Fig. 9). The tympanic isthmus is the only channel for mastoid ventilation in many patients and its blockage **(Fig. 10)** results in a poorly ventilated and developed mastoid cavity in conjunction with isolated disease within the attic but spares the mesotympanum **(Fig. 11)**. A similar clinical presentation occurs in patients with obstruction of the ventilation pathways of the Prussak space **(Fig. 12)** but with different radiological findings showing a reasonably well-ventilated and well-developed mastoid **(Fig. 13)** cavity but extensive attic and possible tympanic cavity disease spread through the posterior pouch of Tröltsch, which is the route of ventilation of the Prussak space **(Fig. 14)**.

- In the presence of epitympanic cholesteatoma and a spared mesotympanum, a distinction should be made between lower epitympanic (Prussak space) disease and upper epitympanic compartment disease based on CT findings.

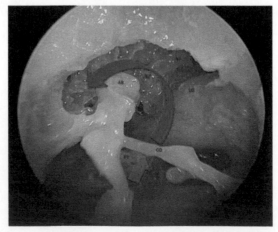

Fig. 7. The ventilation route (*blue arrows*) for the true attic starts with the tympanic isthmus and then moves medially to ventilate the mastoid (posteriorly) and the attic (superiorly). AA, aditus; AS, articulating surface for incus; CD, chorda tympani; LC, lateral semicircular canal; TT, tendon of tensor tympani.

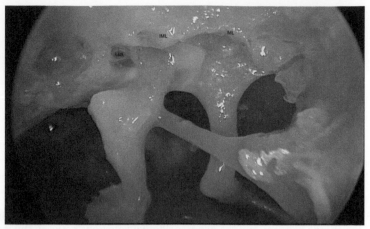

Fig. 8. Left ear: The straight insertion line of the lateral incudomallear ligament (IML) and the downward sloping insertion line of the lateral mallear ligament (LML).

MEASURING THE OPENING PRESSURE OF THE EUSTACHIAN TUBE PREOPERATIVELY

A healthy eustachian tube has been shown to have an opening pressure of around 150 mm H_2O.[10] A blocked eustachian tube usually requires more than 350 mm H_2O. When applying passive pressure through an open perforation, the initial opening pressure is usually significantly higher than any further measurements taking place immediately thereafter. This finding is thought to be related to the surface tension of the mucosal surfaces of the eustachian tube. Asking the patient to actively swallow after a series of measurements usually returns the patient to the initial higher measurement of the opening pressure. This pattern of change in the opening pressures is used to confirm that the measurements obtained are real and that they reflect an opening pressure rather than leakage of air because of inadequate seal. Measurements are obtained clinically by using the setup in (**Fig. 15**), which consist of an endotracheal cuff measuring pump, and a number 8 Foley catheter with both ends cut to allow fitting to the measuring pump and the ear canal. The same procedure is usually performed

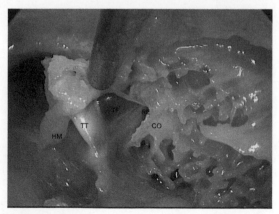

Fig. 9. Left ear: The straight insertion line of the lateral IML and the downward sloping insertion line of the LML. CO, the COG; HM, handle of malleus; TT, tendon of tensor tympani; TF, tensor fold; RE, the recess formed through the insertion of the fold anterior to the COG.

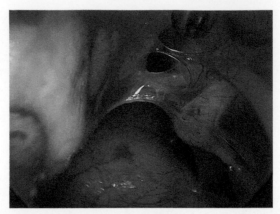

Fig. 10. Blockage of the isthmus. Note the thick fibrous tissue that is closing the isthmus and pulling in the chorda tympani, and the minor incidental adhesions between the incudostapedial joint and the handle of malleus.

during endoscopic transcanal ear surgery, as seen in Video 2. This procedure should not be done in traditional surgery with exposure of dura, sigmoid, and other vascular structures in order to avoid infusing air intracranially.[11]

- Opening pressure measurement is helpful in determining the presence of anatomic obstruction. The initial measurement is always higher than measurements obtained immediately after. An opening pressure greater than 50 cm H_2O denotes anatomic obstruction.

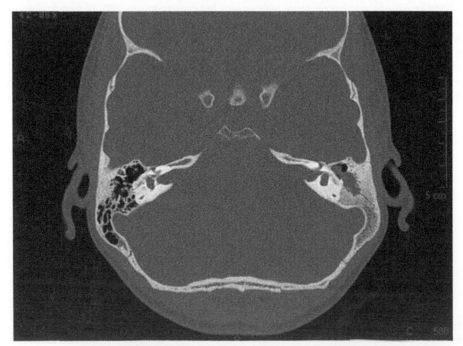

Fig. 11. CT findings in the same patient as in **Fig. 10** with poorly developed and totally opacified mastoid. The only air is in the retracted area within the attic.

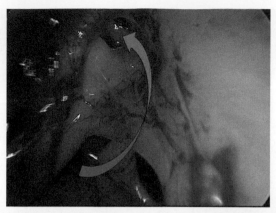

Fig. 12. Left ear after elevation of tympanomeatal flap in a stapes case showing the ventilation pathway (*arrow*) of the Prussak space through the posterior pouch of Tröltsch: the space between the posterior tympanic membrane and a ligamentous fold that joins the posterior spine, the chorda tympani, and the posterior mallear ligament.

VISUAL INTRAOPERATIVE INSPECTION OF THE PROTYMPANIC SPACE

Endoscopic technique allows visualization of the protympanic segment of the eustachian tube. Using a 3-mm, 30° endoscope and introducing it into the superior anterior quadrant of the tympanic membrane, the opening of the cartilaginous tube into the protympanic bony eustachian tube can be identified as a vertical slit opening on top of a cufflike protrusion of the tube into the protympanum/bony eustachian tube, as seen in **Fig. 16.**

Case Discussion

A 22-year-old patient presented to our clinic 8 years ago with right-sided tympanic perforation and underwent endoscopic tympanoplasty without inspection of protympanum. The patient's eardrum healed on 2-month follow-up and he was discharged

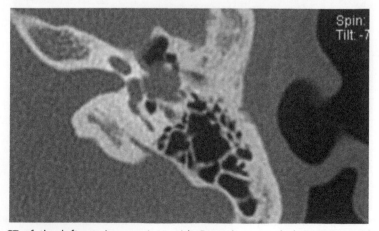

Fig. 13. CT of the left ear in a patient with Prussak space cholesteatoma with a well-ventilated and well-developed mastoid cavity. (*Courtesy of* Dan Lee, MD, Boston, MA.)

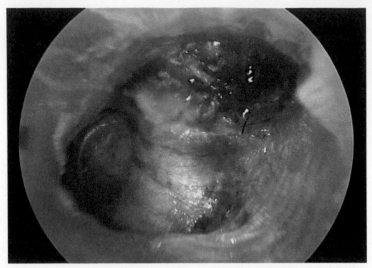

Fig. 14. Same patient as in **Fig. 13.** Endoscopic findings of Prussak space spreading to the mesotympanum through the posterior pouch of Tröltsch, the ventilation route of the Prussak space. (*Courtesy of* Dan Lee, MD, Boston, MA.)

from our care. The patient had returned to his country for many years and presented to us again 6 years after the initial surgery with a history of reperforation that occurred after an upper respiratory infection almost 1 year after the operation. He was taken to the operating room for revision tympanoplasty. Endoscopic examination of the protympanum using the 30° endoscope showed complete obstruction of the eustachian

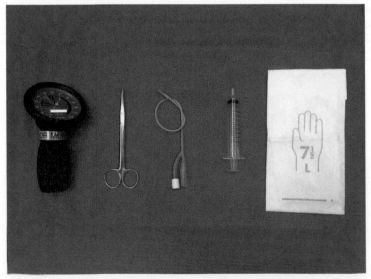

Fig. 15. The setup for measuring the opening pressure of the eustachian tube. The sealing of the ear is performed with a number 8 Foley catheter and pressure is applied using an endotracheal tube cuff pressure monitoring device.

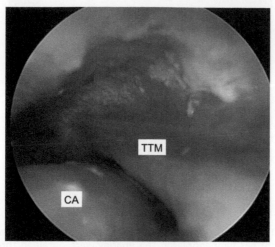

Fig. 16. The opening of the cartilaginous tube into the bony segment/protympanum. Note the vertical slit opening on top of the protruding cufflike proximal end of the cartilaginous tube. CA, carotid artery; TTM, tensor tympani muscle.

tube (**Fig. 17**). This obstruction correlated with the Valsalva CT that had been done preoperatively (**Fig. 18**).

MANAGEMENT ALGORITHM

Fig. 19 shows an algorithm for evaluation of the ventilation of the middle ear cleft based on combination of all the methods discussed earlier. Note that a more upstream ventilation failure in the distal or proximal eustachian tube can incur secondary segmental disease secondary to retraction, medialization of ossicular chain, and inflammatory webbing and stenosis. Therefore, it is important to assess the status of

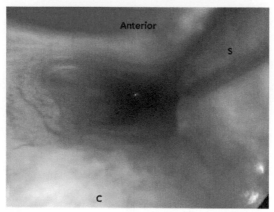

Fig. 17. Right ear: Intraoperative view of the obstructed opening of the eustachian tube in the protympanum in the patient shown in **Fig. 1** who had an earlier successful medial graft tympanoplasty done by the senior author (MT) 8 years earlier. He then reperforated and underwent a revision surgery, during which these images were obtained.

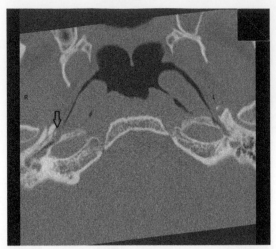

Fig. 18. Valsalva CT of the eustachian tubes of a patient who presented with reperforation after an earlier right ear tympanoplasty. The images were obtained through multiplanar reconstruction in an axial plane that is tilted forward to visualize the whole length of the eustachian tube. Arrow indicates possible site of an obstruction in the protympanic segment on the right side and a patent tubes distally. L, left; R, right.

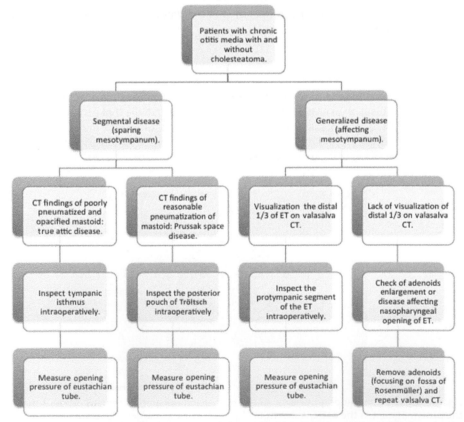

Fig. 19. An algorithm for the assessment of the eustachian tube in patients with chronic ear disease.

the eustachian tube even in the presence of segmental disease with normal-looking mesotympanum.

SUPPLEMENTARY DATA

Supplementary data related to this article can be found at http://dx.doi.org/10.1016/j.otc.2016.05.004.

REFERENCES

1. Linstrom CJ, Silverman CA, Rosen A, et al. Eustachian tube endoscopy in patients with chronic ear disease. Laryngoscope 2000;110:1884–9.
2. Sato H, Hajime N, Iwao H, et al. Eustachian tube function in tympanoplasty. Acta Otolaryngol 1990;110:9–12.
3. Todd NW. There are no accurate tests for eustachian tube function. Arch Otolaryngol Head Neck Surg 2000;126:1041–2.
4. Holmquist J. "Eustachian tube evaluation," acoustic impedance and admittance - the measurement of middle ear function. In: Feldman A, Wilber L, editors. Williams and Wilkins; 1976.
5. Tarabichi M, Najmi M. Site of eustachian tube obstruction in chronic ear disease. Laryngoscope 2015;125(11):2572–5.
6. Palva T, Johnsson L. Epitympanic compartment surgical considerations: reevaluation. Am J Otol 1995;16:505–13.
7. Leuwer R, Schubert R, Kucinski T. Muscular compliance of the auditory tube. A model based survey. Laryngoscope 2002;112:1791–5.
8. Elner A, Ingelstedt S, Ivarsson A. The normal function of the eustachian tube. Acta Otolaryngol 1971;72:320–8.
9. Tarabichi M, Najmi M. Visualization of eustachian tube lumen with Valsalva CT. Laryngoscope 2015;125(3):724–9.
10. Moon JB, Swanson SA. Passive eustachian tube opening pressure – its measurement, normal values, and clinical implications. Arch Otolaryngol 1983;109(6):364–8.
11. Finsnes KA. Lethal intracranial complication following air insufflation with a pneumatic otoscope. Acta Otolaryngol 1973;75:436–8.

The Role of Transtympanic Dilatation of the Eustachian Tube During Chronic Ear Surgery

CrossMark

Muaaz Tarabichi, MD*, Mustafa Kapadia, MD

KEYWORDS

- Eustachian tube obstruction • Cholesteatoma • Tympanic perforation
- Tympanoplasty • CT of temporal bone • Valsalva maneuver • Balloon dilatation
- Eustachian tuboplasty

KEY POINTS

- The proximal cartilaginous eustachian tube is the most common site of anatomic obstruction in chronic otitis media.
- Access to that area is provided for inspection and intervention through the transtympanic route using a 30° angled endoscope.
- The carotid canal can be identified endoscopically and the anatomy of the protympanum is variable.
- The protympanum is the only area of the eustachian tube with close proximity to the carotid, and safe endoscopic access to the proximal cartilaginous tube is possible beyond this dangerous segment.
- Dilatation of the proximal segment of the eustachian tube is safely undertaken through the transtympanic route during chronic ear surgery after visualization of the carotid canal.

 Video content accompanies this article at http://www.oto.theclinics.com.

INTRODUCTION

Balloon dilatation of the eustachian tube has been reported with a significant degree of success and patient safety.[1] Instrumentation of the eustachian tube is performed by introducing the balloon catheter through the nasopharyngeal opening of the tube and subsequently dilating the cartilaginous segment of the tube.[2] Safety consideration with regard to avoiding possible injury to the carotid artery has limited the area of

Financial Disclosures: None.

Conflict of Interest: None.

Department of Otolaryngology, American Hospital Dubai, PO Box 5566, Oud Mehta Road, Dubai, United Arab Emirates

* Corresponding author.

E-mail address: mtarabichi@ahdubai.com

oto.theclinics.com

instrumentation to the distal end of the tube, which is probably the least likely obstructed segment. Other sites of obstruction in the proximal area of the eustachian tube have been reported in patients undergoing chronic ear surgery.[3] Endoscopic ear surgery allows access to and visualization of the protympanic segment of the eustachian tube, including the carotid canal.[4] Transtympanic introduction of the balloon catheter beyond the carotid canal into the cartilaginous eustachian tube ensures the safety of the dilatation along with the dilatation coverage of a wider segment of the cartilaginous tube.[5]

Technique

All patients undergoing surgery for chronic otitis media (perforations/cholesteatoma/retraction/drainage) should be assessed for the source of ventilation failure as per the previous article. Intraoperatively, a measurement of the opening pressure of the eustachian tube is performed up to 50 cm of water using the setup in **Fig. 1**. If the air pressure is not released through the eustachian tube at 50 cm of water, then endoscopic evaluation of the protympanic segment of the eustachian tube is performed using a 30°, 3-mm, 15-cm rigid endoscope that is introduced anterior to the handle of malleus after detaching the tympanic membrane remnant from the handle of the malleus.

- Evidence of obstruction in the proximal cartilaginous tube is required before proceeding with transtympanic dilatation. It is usually a combination of Valsalva computed tomography (CT) showing open distal tube and inability to open up the tube at 50 cm of water or direct endoscopic evidence of blockage.

The protympanic segment is then assessed for clear impression of the carotid artery canal, presence of blind pouches, and for evidence of obstruction beyond that (**Fig. 2**). An eustachian tube balloon dilatation catheter (Spiggle & Theis, Germany) is used. The catheter is usually shipped with a metal stylet that runs within the catheter.

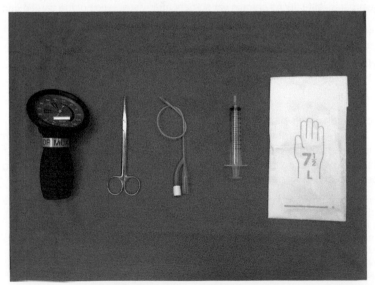

Fig. 1. The setup for measuring opening pressure of the eustachian tube. The sealing of the ear is performed with a number 8 Foley catheter and application of pressure is done by an endotracheal tube cuff pressure monitoring device.

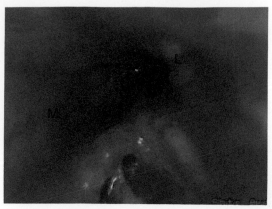

Fig. 2. Right ear: View of the obstructed protympanic segment of the eustachian tube. L, Lateral; M, Medial.

A 30° deflection is bent at the distal 1 cm of the stylet. The proximal end of the stylet is looped to allow for rotating and orienting the deflection at the distal end toward the opening of the eustachian tube (**Fig. 3**). The stylet functions like a guidewire and the catheter is fed into the eustachian tube over the stylet until it is well within the distal tube. The stylet is then removed. Then the balloon is inflated by infusing saline to 10 cmH$_2$O as indicated by the inflating device. At this point, the catheter should be easily moving within the eustachian tube because the distal end of the tube is much larger than the inflated balloon catheter. Then, with the balloon inflated, the catheter is pulled out until it is lodged at the isthmus, which is much smaller than the inflated balloon catheter and does not allow it to be pulled out. Then the balloon is deflated and pulled by 0.5 cm and inflation is performed again. Given the V shape of the tube, the surgeon experiences catheter pull-in to the nasopharynx as it is inflated. This pull-in confirms to the surgeon that it is located within the eustachian tube (**Fig. 4**).

- The presence of catheter pull is a clear evidence of cannulating the eustachian tube. It happens because of the V-like shape of the tube with the distal segment being much larger than the proximal part. It also confirms that the distal segment is not involved in the obstruction.

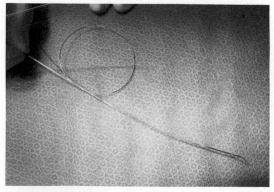

Fig. 3. The stylet is angled at its distal end and the proximal end is looped so it can be rotated to direct the distal end angled tip orientation to help direct the catheter toward the opening of the eustachian tube.

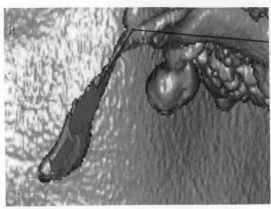

Fig. 4. Three-dimensional reconstruction of the airspaces in the temporal bone in a Valsalva CT showing the V-like shape of the eustachian tube, and the catheter pull-in that happens when the balloon is inflated.

The catheter is then pulled out until the balloon area is barely visualized using the 30° scope. Another approach is to pull the tube in small increments and attempt inflation of balloon, checking for the point where the balloon is lodged and stable within the isthmus without the need to hold on to keep it from advancing as it is being inflated (**Fig. 5**).

- The lodging of the tube and the lack of catheter pull as the catheter is pulled out confirms that the balloon is engaging the isthmus of the eustachian tube.

The pressure is maintained at 10 bar for 2 minutes and then deflated and pulled out. Reinspection of the area with a 3-mm 30° endoscope is performed to assess for change of aperture of the eustachian tube in that area (**Fig. 6**). Then the opening pressure is tested again to verify its decrease beyond 50 cm of water. Video 1 shows the procedure.

Case study
This involves a woman who presented with chronically discharging ear. Multiple attempts at local treatments with combinations of steroid and antibiotic ear drops

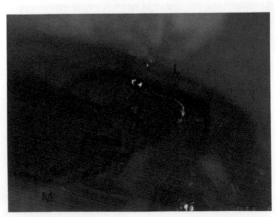

Fig. 5. Right ear: Balloon dilatation of the eustachian tube using a balloon catheter.

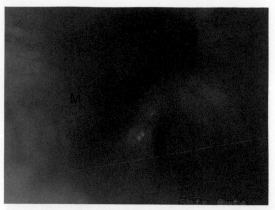

Fig. 6. Right ear: Postdilatation view of the protympanic segment of the eustachian tube; the downward and anterior turn of the tube can now be visualized.

were made without any response (Video 2). Valsalva CT was performed and showed visualization of the whole length of the eustachian tube on the right and patent distal eustachian tube on the left with obstruction of the proximal cartilaginous segment (**Figs. 7** and **8**). The patient had exploration of the ear, which showed intact ossicular chain, no cholesteatoma, granulation tissue posteriorly and anteriorly, and thick mucus. Transtympanic balloon dilatation was performed with simple tympanoplasty. Postoperatively the patient did well and the eardrum healed with no discharge and normal hearing. Valsalva CT was performed 3 months postprocedure and showed visualization of the whole length of the eustachian tube on the left side (**Figs. 9** and **10**).

Anatomic Considerations: Relationship of the Carotid to the Eustachian Tube

Given the limited microscopic access to the protympanum, it has been the common wisdom in the otology community to avoid any interventions involving the proximal

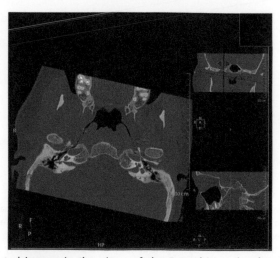

Fig. 7. Reconstructed images in the plane of the Eustachian tube showing dilated distal tube on both sides and obstructed proximal cartilaginous tube on the left side (*red arrow*).

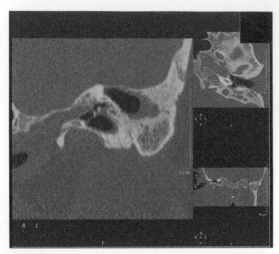

Fig. 8. Parasagittal reconstruction in the plane of the eustachian tube in the same patient and CT images as in **Fig. 7**.

eustachian tube. Further confirmation of that close relationship is found on the axial plane CT images, in which the carotid is very prominent and appears in close proximity to the whole length of the eustachian tube (**Fig. 11**). However, all of the cartilaginous tube is well away from the carotid artery because it turns downward toward the nasopharynx (see **Fig. 9**). **Fig. 12** shows a parasagittal multiplanar reconstruction of the CT taken in the plane of the eustachian tube defining the downward slope of the cartilaginous tube. **Fig. 13** is the same image as **Fig. 12** but with an overlay of the carotid artery course obtained from a parallel section just medial to **Fig. 12**. It confirms that the carotid artery takes a different direction and intersects with only a limited segment of the medial aspect of the protympanic bony segment of the tube. If the protympanic segment is visualized endoscopically and instrumentation is directed anterior to it, carotid artery safety should be ensured.

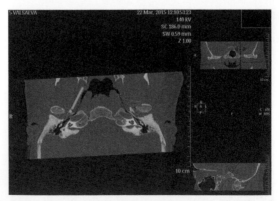

Fig. 9. CT done 3 months post dilatation of the same patient in **Fig. 7**. Reconstructed images in the plane of the Eustachian tube showing visualization of the whole length of the tube on the left side (*red arrow*, the same area is seen obstructed in **Fig. 7** pre dilatation). Note that on the Right side the whole cartilaginous tube and part of the bony segment are well clear of carotid (*green line*) and the carotid proximity to the Eustachian tube is limited to a certain area within the bony part (*red line*).

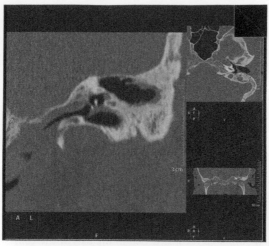

Fig. 10. Parasagittal reconstruction in the plane of the eustachian tube in the same patient and CT images as in **Fig. 9**.

- Contrary to common perception, the carotid only engages the eustachian tube in a limited segment of the posterior protympanum. The whole cartilaginous tube slopes downward away from the carotid anatomically.

Anatomic Considerations: Anatomy of Protympanum

The lack of access to the protympanum has resulted in a distorted view of the anatomy of the eustachian tube. For endoscopic observers of that area, the idea of a bony eustachian tube seems to be counterintuitive. The existing definition of the bony eustachian tube is based on lack of access when using the microscope. Once visualized with the 30° scope, that part of the anatomy ceases to be an eustachian tube and becomes just an anterior extension of the mesotympanum, or the anterior part of the protympanum. The proximal cartilaginous tube opens up into that bony extension of the mesotympanum in a similar way that the distal end opens up into the nasopharynx: with a cufflike protrusion of the tube with an opening in the middle of that cuff (**Fig. 14**).

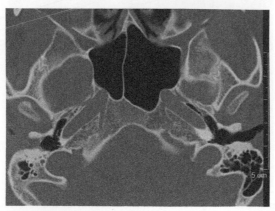

Fig. 11. Axial CT of the protympanum showing that much of the medial wall of the tube is occupied by the carotid artery.

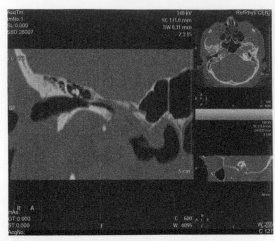

Fig. 12. Parasagittal multiplanar reconstruction in the axis of the tube showing the downward orientation of the cartilaginous tube.

- The common orthodoxy of a bony and cartilaginous tube does not stand up to endoscopic inspection. The bony tube is part of the protympanum and the cartilaginous part is the whole eustachian tube.

The main source of variation of the anatomy comes from pneumatization of an air cell medial to the carotid artery or between the carotid and the tensor tympani muscle encasement. This pneumatization results in a blind false passage that might lead observers to mistake it for the eustachian tube (**Fig. 15**). However, on further and deeper introduction of the scope, the eustachian tube can be identified as the most lateral opening in the anterior protympanum. The most demanding part of the technique is to make the angle between the ear canal and the eustachian tube and to avoid catheterization of the more medial blind pouch formed by the pneumatization of the bone medial to the carotid.

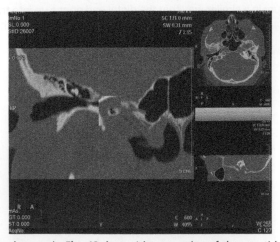

Fig. 13. The same plane as in **Fig. 12**, but with an overlay of the carotid artery course obtained from another image parallel to the one showed in **Fig. 12** but more medial to show the carotid.

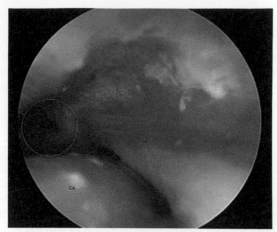

Fig. 14. Left ear: Looking at the protympanum with a 3-mm 30° scope. The proximal carti- laginous tube opens up into the bony extension of the mesotympanum in a similar way to how the distal end opens up into the nasopharynx: with a cufflike protrusion of the tube with an opening in the middle area of that cuff (*blue circle*). CA, carotid; TTM, tensor tympani muscle.

Safety Considerations

There are 2 main safety concerns in transtympanic eustachian tube dilatation:

1. Ossicular chain: more specifically the possible coiling of the catheter in the middle ear and the medial displacement/dislocation of the handle of malleus. This outcome can be avoided by continuous endoscopic monitoring of the advancing catheter. Clinicians should always consider aborting the procedure if the catheter is meeting too much resistance. Maintaining the introducer in position while advancing the catheter over it also prevents coiling in the middle ear. Damage to the stapes can be avoided by correctly introducing the catheter from the superior posterior aspect of the ear canal rather than more inferiorly. This technique also serves to align the catheter with the anatomy and orientation of the eustachian tube.

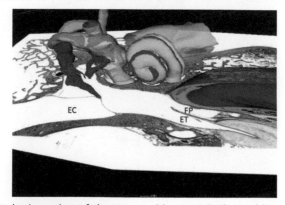

Fig. 15. Axial histologic section of the temporal bone with the cochlea and malleus simu- lated for orientation. Note the pneumatization and formation of a medial false passage. EC, external auditory canal; ET, eustachian tube; FP, false passage.

2. Carotid artery: inspection of the protympanum for the carotid canal and any dehiscence is an important first step in ensuring the safety of this procedure. Directing the catheter anterior to the carotid and inferiorly away from it, is essential to be able to intubate the tube with the catheter. Atraumatic insertion with measured application of pressure is the third requirement. The procedure discussed earlier allows the surgeon to confirm the presence of the catheter in the right position before inflating the balloon.

RESULTS

Transtympanic dilatation of the tube is a safe and atraumatic intervention. In more than 100 dilatation procedures performed by the author, there were almost no bleeding or mucosal lacerations evident on immediate inspection of the protympanum and the dilated proximal segment. There were no carotid-related complications despite the presence of dehiscence in 2 cases. In 3 ears, the procedure was aborted because of the inability to push the catheter through. The aperture of the visualized tube was consistently larger than predilatation in every case in which catheter placement and dilatation were done. The opening pressure was consistently less after dilatation in all but 1 patient who had persistent failure to open the eustachian tube after dilatation. In 9 patients, postdilatation CT was obtained 3 to 4 months after procedure and evidence of increased patency in the protympanic area was observed (**Figs. 16** and **17**).

- Transtympanic dilatation is a safe but technically demanding procedure that has significant anecdotal evidence of efficacy.

DISCUSSION

Chronic ear surgery has always involved removing disease and regaining function without much attention to the pathophysiologic process underlying the disease. Because many of the obstruction sites lie out of reach of traditional instruments, it is always assumed that time and age have resolved any obstruction.[3] Failures in chronic ear surgery have been shown to correlate with persistent eustachian tube dysfunction.[6] The preponderance of reported evidence indicates that the cartilaginous tube and its distal segment harbor most of the sites of obstruction.[7-9] However, Linstrom and colleagues[3] described their experience in using fiberoptic flexible miniscopes introduced through the ear during chronic ear surgery to evaluate the patency

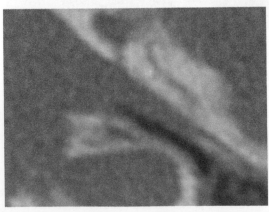

Fig. 16. Preoperative CT of the protympanic segment of the eustachian tube.

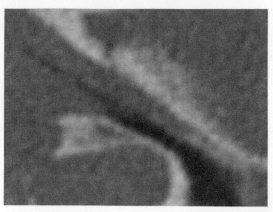

Fig. 17. Postoperative CT of the protympanic segment in the same patient at 3 months from intervention.

of the eustachian tube. Their results indicated that much of the obstruction existed in the protympanic segment of the eustachian tube. They also found that, in cases in which the obstruction can be bypassed, the obstructed segment did not extend much beyond that point. However, the quality of the images obtained with the fiber-optic device they used is limited, which can lead to misleading assessment of these images. Endoscopic ear surgery with rigid scopes allows the high-resolution evaluation and instrumentation of the protympanic segment of the tube.[4] The authors have reproduced the Lindstrom and colleagues[3] study using high-resolution rigid scopes and Valsalva CT and have confirmed their findings in our patient population: the distal tube is patent and the proximal part is the site of the obstruction in chronic ear disease.[10] This area contains the isthmus, the narrowest segment of the cartilaginous tube, and is in close proximity to the tympanic cavity and any recurrent inflammatory process within it during childhood years. However, there is a degree of variability in the site of obstruction and some of our patients have obstruction in other more distal locations in the eustachian tube.

Recently, balloon dilatation of the eustachian tube has been described with significant degree of success. The procedure is designed to address obstruction located in the distal segment of the cartilaginous segment in proximity to the nasopharyngeal opening of the eustachian tube.[1,2] The procedure is performed by introducing a balloon dilatation catheter through the nasopharyngeal opening of the tube with design features that prevent its introduction to the area of the carotid artery canal. The procedure and the catheters are designed to stay clear of the protympanic segment of the tube, an area that, in the authors' opinion, represents the most common site of anatomic obstruction of the eustachian tube.

The term protympanic segment of the eustachian tube is nonspecific and is a misrepresentation of the anatomy. It is hard to make a distinction between that and the bony eustachian tube. It is more sensible to think of this area as an extension of the mesotympanum anteriorly, and it should be called the protympanum. It can be divided into 2 areas: the area medial to the carotid canal and the area anterior to that. The carotid canal is uniformly identifiable by expert inspection of the protympanic segment (see **Fig. 15**). In most cases, the cartilaginous tube opens up into this space with a cufflike structure very similar to the nasopharyngeal opening of the tube. The term eustachian tube should apply only to the cartilaginous tube linking the nasopharynx to the protympanum. This definition is contrary to the common ortho-doxy of the bony part of the eustachian tube but it better reflects the anatomy as seen by the endoscope.

Endoscopic ear surgery with rigid straight-view and angled-view scopes allows wide-view visualization of the tympanic cavity, especially anteriorly.[11] Further expo-sure anteriorly into the protympanic part of the eustachian tube can be obtained with a 30° 3-mm endoscope, which allows the visualization of much of the bony segment and a significant part of the cartilaginous segment as it turns inferiorly and medially at almost 120° to the bony segment.[12] This visualization depends on the abil-ity to introduce the endoscope anterior to the handle of the malleus. Access can also be obtained even with an intact tympanic membrane anteriorly by separating the membrane from the handle of the malleus and lifting it up anteriorly against the anterior ear canal. It has been a consistent finding that the postdilatation picture was different, with clear widening of the aperture of that segment compared with the predilatation findings, confirming the cartilaginous nature of that segment anterior to the carotid ca-nal. The safety of the carotid and its canal can be ascertained from the consistency of the identification of the carotid canal in the medial wall of the protympanum that was observed here and the introduction of the balloon catheter beyond that point as well as the different steps in the techniques outlined earlier to confirm the catheter location within the eustachian tube.

The anatomy of the protympanic segment of the eustachian tube is variable and a clear understanding of that anatomy and full visualization are preconditions to safe instrumentation of the proximal end of the eustachian tube. In about 30% of the ears examined, there was a pneumatization of the area anterior to the carotid, which resulted in a ridge of bone that divided the protympanic opening of the eustachian tube into a lateral opening for the eustachian tube and a medial false passage (see **Fig. 15**). This variability requires the surgeon to introduce a small scope far enough anteriorly to determine the exact anatomy of that area (**Figs. 18** and **19**). If the false passage is cannulated, and if the surgeon fails to clearly identify the carotid canal and to ascertain the intubation of the eustachian tube anterior to the canal, there is the possibility of damaging the carotid canal (see **Fig. 15**).

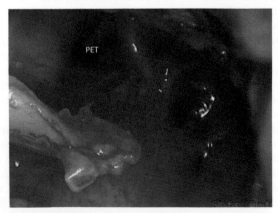

Fig. 18. Right ear: The protympanum is visualized after lifting of the tympanic membrane off the handle of the malleus. An apparent opening of the eustachian tube is visualized. PET, protympanic eustachian tube.

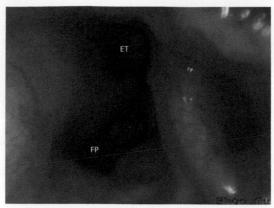

Fig. 19. Further introduction of the scope shows the true opening of the eustachian tube laterally to a false passage that was initially thought to be the opening of the tube.

Multiplanar reconstruction of high-resolution CT images of the temporal bone has allowed the orientation of the sections in the plane of the eustachian tube and the ability to bring it to view.

Most otologists have taken to studying the axial and coronal CT images of the temporal bone. On axial cuts through the protympanum and the carotid artery, careful study of these images in the axis of the tube results in better understanding of the anatomy of the proximal segment. Preoperative CT is common practice in cholesteatoma surgery and careful attention to the eustachian tube anatomy and disorder should be part of any preoperative assessment of these patients.

SUMMARY

Endoscopic technique allows visualization of the protympanic segment of the eustachian tube in patients undergoing chronic ear surgery. Balloon dilatation of the area can be undertaken with clear widening of the obstructed areas.

SUPPLEMENTARY DATA

Supplementary data related to this article can be found at http://dx.doi.org/10.1016/j.otc.2016.05.013.

REFERENCES

1. Poe DS, Juha S, Ilmari P. Balloon dilation of the cartilaginous eustachian tube. Otolaryngol Head Neck Surg 2011;144(4):563–9.
2. Ockermann T, Ulf R, Tahwinder U, et al. Balloon dilatation eustachian tuboplasty: a clinical study. Laryngoscope 2010;120:1411–6.
3. Linstrom CJ, Carol AS, Arie R, et al. Eustachian tube endoscopy in patients with chronic ear disease. Laryngoscope 2000;110:1884–9.
4. Tarabichi M. Transcanal endoscopic management of cholesteatoma. Otol Neurotol 2010;31:580–8.
5. Tarabichi M, Najmi M. Transtympanic dilatation of the eustachian tube during chronic ear surgery. Acta Otolaryngol 2015;135(7):640–4.
6. Sato H, Hajime N, Iwao H, et al. Eustachian tube function in tympanoplasty. Acta Otolaryngol 1990;110:9–12.

7. Takahashi H, Fujita A, Honjo I. Site of eustachian tube dysfunction in patients with otitis media with effusion. Am J Otolaryngol 1987;8:361–3.
8. Edelstein DR, Magnan J, Parisier C. Microfiberoptic evaluation of the middle ear cavity. Am J Otol 1994;15:50.
9. Takahashi H, Honjo I, Fujita A. Endoscopic findings at the pharyngeal orifice of the eustachian tube in otitis media with effusion. Eur Arch Otorhinolaryngol 1996;253:42–7.
10. Tarabichi M, Najmi M. Site of eustachian tube obstruction in chronic ear disease. Laryngoscope 2015;125(11):2572–5.
11. Tarabichi M. Endoscopic management of limited attic cholesteatoma. Laryngoscope 2004;114:1157–62.
12. Graves GO, Edwards LF. The eustachian tube: review of its descriptive, microscopic, topographic, and clinical anatomy. Arch Otolaryngol 1944;39:359–97.

Transnasal Endoscopic Eustachian Tube Surgery

Marc Dean, MD[a,b],*, Timothy Lian, MD, MBA, FACS[a]

KEYWORDS

- Patulous eustachian tube • Eustachian tube dysfunction • Eustachian tube dilation

KEY POINTS

- Shim placement should be considered as first-line surgical treatment of patulous Eustachian dysfunction, as it is well tolerated, has a low morbidity, and is reversible.
- Injection of fillers, such as calcium hydroxyapatite, should be reserved as salvage procedures after soft tissue augmentation in patulous dysfunction of the Eustachian tube due to it tendency to migrate and transitory effect.
- Balloon dilation of the cartilaginous Eustachian tube is a feasible alternative to tympanostomy tube placement in patients with long-standing, refractory dilatory dysfunction.
- Balloon dilation improves Eustachian tube function via deep muscle stretch, dermabrasion of the diseased mucosal epithelium, and selective scarring of the submucosa.
- Management of any underlying pathophysiology, such as allergies or reflux, is necessary for long-term success in patients with dilatory dysfunction.

 Video content accompanies this article at http://www.oto.theclinics.com.

INTRODUCTION

The Eustachian tube (ET) is a dynamic structure that has long plagued both physicians and patients alike. It has traditionally been classified as a part of the auditory system, in part, due to its importance in regulating middle ear pressures but also because manifestations of ET dysfunction (ETD) tend to be otologic in nature. Recent investigations have found that a large majority of ET derangements occur in the nasopharyngeal portion of ET and are more rhinologic in nature.[1] This unique dichotomy has led to speculation and confusion regarding the function and physiology of the ET since was first mentioned by Aristotle in the fourth century BC. It was not until the advent

Disclosures: Consultant for Acclarent (M. Dean); none (T. Lian).
[a] Department of Otolaryngology-Head and Neck Surgery, Louisiana State University Health Sciences Center - Shreveport, Shreveport, LA, USA; [b] Otorhinologic Research Institute, Fort Worth, TX, USA
* Corresponding author. Department of Otolaryngology-Head and Neck Surgery, Louisiana State University Health Sciences Center - Shreveport, Shreveport, LA.
E-mail address: marc.dean@gmail.com

of fiberoptic endoscopy in the late twentieth century that the dynamic nature of the ET was first postulated.[2] It is now clear that the ET functions to regulate middle ear pressure with respect to atmosphere pressure, facilitate clearance of middle ear secretions, and protect the middle ear from sound and accumulation of nasopharyngeal secretions.[3] Although the function and nature of the ET has remained elusive until recently, the anatomy of the ET is much more concrete. The composition of the tube itself was first described by Bartolomeus Eustachius in 1562, and muscular attachments were further defined by Antonio Valsalva in 1704.[2] The adult ET has a reported length of 31 mm to 38 mm, of which approximately the medial two-thirds is lined with fibrocartilage and the lateral osseous one-third is within the temporal bone. Three-dimensional modeling has demonstrated an hourglass–like central constriction, referred to as the isthmus, near the junction of these segments. The cartilaginous portion is obliquely angled approximately 45°, and is composed of anterior and posterior laminae. The anterior lamina provides an insertion for the tensor veli palatine muscle approximately 12 to 20 mm deep to the pharyngeal orifice, resulting in a dynamic valvelike region. The constriction of the tensor veli palatine initiates a coordinated sequence in concert with the other peritubal muscles, which leads to the valvelike opening and closing of the ET. This process occurs in 4 distinct phases lasting less than half a second. The abnormal closure of this valve is believed to be the underlying factor in ETD.[4]

Despite a definitive anatomic description of the ET, its elusive nature combined with its remote location in the nasopharynx, has resulted in a lack of objective diagnostic tools and therapeutic treatments. Recent advances in both endoscopic techniques and diagnostic tools have brought a renewed interest restoring the function of ET via therapeutic interventions. The past 2 decades have seen a renewed interest in the surgical management of the ET disorders fueled by the adaptation of modern rhinologic techniques related to traditional ET procedures. As the understanding of both the dynamic and anatomic nature of the ET has increased, so have the options for management. The current surgical treatments available for dilatory dysfunction have expanded from the traditional adenoidectomy and myringotomy with tube placement to include laser and microdebrider Eustachian tuboplasty, as well as balloon dilation of the ET. The surgical corrections for patulous dysfunction have evolved to include, injection of calcium hydroxyapatite, shim placement, and soft tissue augmentation.[5] The purpose of this article is to give an updated review for the evaluation and diagnosis of a dysfunctional ET, as well as describe the current surgical interventions available for the treatment ETD.

CONTENT/DISCUSSION

ETD is defined by symptoms and signs of pressure dysregulation in the middle ear, and until recently there were many varied definitions of what this meant clinically. A recent consensus statement has clarified and standardized the definition. It divides ETD into 3 subtypes: baro-challenge-induced, dilatory, and patulous dysfunction. Dilatory dysfunction can be further broken down as follows: functional obstruction, dynamic dysfunction (muscular failure), and anatomic obstruction[6] Baro-challenge dysfunction is elicited or exacerbated by changes in altitude or barometric pressure. Dilatory dysfunction of the ET is characterized as aural fullness that is usually associated with some degree of hearing loss or tinnitus. When it becomes more severe, otalgia followed by otitis media and the complications of otitis, such as atelectasis, retraction pockets, or even cholesteatoma. Dilatory dysfunction has been estimated to affect up to 30% to 80% of children at some point during their childhood.[7] Despite the maturation of the ET, and the aggressive medical and surgical management of underlying pathologies, ETD continues to plague approximately 1% of the population throughout their adult lives.[8] In 1997, Kujawaski ushered in the modern era of surgical treatment of the ET by describing the first tuboplasty. He approached the ET both transoral as well as transnasal to obliterate both mucosa and cartilage from the posterior cushion using a laser. Ten years later, Metson described a rhinologic-based version of this procedure that used a microdebrider through an exclusively transnasal approach. In 2010, Ockerman[2] published his study exploring the value in using sinus balloons as a potential surgical intervention for the treatment of ETD.

As more physicians contemplate the surgical correction of dilatory and baro-challenge dysfunction, it is important to have a good understanding of patulous dysfunction, as it can result from overcorrection of dilatory dysfunction as well as mimic dilatory dysfunction to the less-experienced clinician. Patients with patulous dysfunction also present with aural fullness and potentially otalgia, but they most often relate a history of autophony, both to voice and to respiratory sounds.[4] Patients with patulous ET may state that their symptoms are better in the supine position, during upper respiratory tract infections, and worse with exercise, public speaking, singing, or caffeine ingestion. Myringotomy and tympanostomy tube placement can alleviate aural fullness and tympanic membrane excursions, but is often ineffective for autophony. A recent systemic review of the published literature by Hussein and colleagues[5] described several transnasal surgical options now being used, including shim placement, augmentation with injectable filler, or autologous tissue.

The treatment of ETD is further confounded by its multifactorial pathophysiology. One study, looking at the possible causes of dilatory dysfunction, found that mucosal edema involving the ET orifice was present in 83% of patients and 74% of patients were noted to have decreased anterolateral wall motion that was attributed to inflammation.[9] Poe reports the most common cause of dilatory dysfunction is mucosal inflammation within the cartilaginous ET, most often secondary to allergic rhinitis, chronic rhinosinusitis, laryngopharyngeal reflux, and smoke exposure. It has also been observed in patients with systemic mucosal disorders, such as granulomatous disease, cystic fibrosis, Sampter triad, and Kartagener syndrome.[4] Patulous dysfunction on the other hand has most often been associated with recent and significant weight loss; however, more recent studies have shown rheumatologic, or other chronic disease conditions, stress, and oral contraceptives to be more likely causes.[10] Identifying and treating these underlying pathologies before invasive therapies will both improve outcomes and avoid unnecessary interventions.

Anatomic abnormalities can also play a role in ET disorders, especially when it is found to be unilateral. For instance, residual adenoid tissue or significant scarring after adenoidectomy has been associated with limitation of tubal opening, and cartilaginous abnormalities of the posteromedial wall have been found to cause obstruction leading to dilatory dysfunction.[9] It is important to mention that if the obstruction is isolated to the inferior portion of the ET it can prop open the superior portion of the tube causing patulous dysfunction. Nasal anatomy may also indirectly contribute to ETD. A study by McNicoll[11] showed in a prospective controlled trial that septoplasty corrected 94% ETD in submariners with septal deviation. These findings indicate nasal airflow may play a significant role in disorders of the ET.

It is the experience of the authors that successful treatment and management of ET disorders is directly related to the accuracy in identifying the pathogenesis related to both the patient's symptoms and the causative factors. This requires a detailed past medical history and physical examination in conjunction with several validated symptom scores and function tests. Obtaining the past medical history needs to be targeted at identifying both underlying causative factors, the timing of symptoms related to certain potential triggers, such as changes in barometric pressure and altitude, as well as the worsening of sinonasal congestion and gastroesophageal reflux disease. The physical examination begins with bilateral otomicroscopy. Patients with active dilatory dysfunction often exhibit tympanic membrane retraction or effusion, but it is important to remember that although retraction pockets in the posterior superior quadrant or attic may have originated from ETD, they may persist or progress because of unrelated inflammatory mechanisms. Nonfixed retraction or atelectasis, or middle ear effusions indicate active dilatory dysfunction, whereas medial and lateral excursions of the tympanic membrane with ipsilateral nasal breathing indicate active patulous dysfunction. If the patient is suspected of having patulous dysfunction by history, having the patient exercise for several minutes before otoscopy may provoke symptoms, if not present initially.[10]

Endoscopic examination of the upper respiratory tract and ET should be performed to evaluate for evidence of inflammatory or granulomatous disease. To optimize the view of the ET orifice during opening and closing, the endoscope should be brought to the tubal orifice and directed 45° laterally and superiorly to the nasal floor. This can be accomplished by rotating a fiberoptic endoscope into position either from the ipsilateral or contralateral nasal cavity.[4] The ET orifice is located just posterior to the inferior turbinate. The torus tubarius or "posterior cushion" contains the mobile medial cartilaginous lamina marking the anterior aspect of the ET. The most common findings seen in dilatory dysfunction include mucosal inflammation, hypertrophy, excessive mucus, hyperemia, and cobble-stoning,[9] although patients with patulous dysfunction often exhibit a concave defect in the anterolateral wall leading to insufficient closure of the lumen as opposed to the normal convex bulge.[10]

As clinicians are beginning to understand the pathophysiology behind ET disorders, there have been many studies looking at both the efficacy and safety of surgical procedures aimed at treating the ET. Several meta-analyses have concluded that although surgical management of the ET has been shown to be relatively safe and patients report significant benefit, there is not enough objective evidence to determine the actual effectiveness and indications of these procedures. This has been attributed, in part, to the lack of validated diagnostic tools and applicable function tests.[12] A large number of tests related to ET function have been created, but unfortunately the clinical relevance of these tests has remained unclear. Compounding this, little to no recognized standards exist regarding evaluation protocols, thus making the current data that have been generated difficult to compare.[13] In 2012, McCoul and colleagues[14] attempted to address this deficiency with the introduction of the eustachian tube dysfunction questionnaire (ETDQ-7), a validated Quality-of-Life Questionnaire, which has been shown to statistically correlate with clinical and objective improvement. It is important to note that although the ETDQ-7 is sensitive and specific in identifying patients with a dysfunctional ET, it is ineffective in differentiating between patulous and dilatory dysfunction.[15] In 2013, Doyle and colleagues[13] performed a randomized controlled trial that identified 4 ET function test parameters (Valsalva, ET opening pressure, dilatory efficiency, and percentage of positive pressure equilibrated) that when looked at together correctly identified patients with ETD with a sensitivity of 95% and a specificity of 83%. Interestingly, the tests evaluating the opening efficiency of the ET where statistically relevant; however, tests evaluating structural properties were not.[13] Impedance tympanometry is the most objective and sensitive test to evaluate patients with patulous dysfunction, as it shows fluctuations in tympanic membrane compliance with ipsilateral nasal breathing while the patient is symptomatic.

It is important to note that although this test is essential to differentiate between dilatory and patulous dysfunction especially with a positive ETDQ-7, it cannot be used in patients with a pressure equalization tube or tympanic membrane perforation.[4] Together these tests are beginning to provide researchers and clinicians with objective and validated metrics that can help evaluate the effectiveness of specific treatments of ETD, and there are now several ongoing prospective randomized trials using these tools to better understand the role specific treatments play in management of ETD.

One of the reasons clinically relevant diagnostic tests have not evolved earlier is due to the paucity of proven treatment options. In fact, current medical management of dilatory ETD is directed at treating the underlying pathology, as there is no Food and Drug Administration–approved therapy indicated for ETD. A placebo-controlled randomized double-blinded trial evaluated intranasal Triamcinolone spray over 6 weeks in patients with otitis media with effusion or negative middle ear pressure failed to show any statistical difference.[16] Medical therapies have been slightly more successful in patients with patulous dysfunction, and they are aimed at thickening peritubal mucosa, reestablishing a competent valve. Medications that stimulate mucus production or tissue inflammation, such as a saturated solution of potassium iodine drops mixed with water or juice taken 3 times, have been used with varied results. Hydrochloric acid–based topical nasal drops, boric acid, silver nitrate, salicylic acid powder, and phenol are all irritants that been used to create mucosal inflammation and increase mucus production. Hormones such as Premarin and Depo-Estradiol estrogens may be used to cause mucosal hypertrophy and provide relief of symptoms for undetermined durations.[4] Although weight loss has been thought to lead to patulous dysfunction, weight gain as treatment for aural symptoms is generally discouraged. When medical management is insufficient to control symptoms secondary to either dilatory or patulous dysfunction, and causes a significant decrease in quality of life, surgical intervention should be considered.

In most cases it is important to obtain a computed tomography (CT) scan before committing to a surgical intervention. The images are helpful for defining the length and diameter of the ET as well as evaluating for internal carotid artery (ICA) dehiscence. However, in a retrospective review, Schoder demonstrated that preoperative high-resolution CT scan of the temporal bone does not seem to be suitable to predict intraoperative or postoperative difficulties of balloon dilation of the ET. Nevertheless, for inexperienced surgeons, or to further investigate unclear pathology such as superior canal dehiscence, CT scans of the temporal bone may beneficial in understanding the relation between ICA and the ET as well as identifying potential obstructing pathology, such as cartilaginous anomalies, or tumors.[17]

Modern endoscopic Eustachian tuboplasty was first introduced less than 20 years ago and remains a satisfactory surgical option to treat pathologies located in the proximal portions of the nasopharyngeal ET orifice and can be efficiently combined with adenoidectomy or sinus surgery. The goal of this procedure is to remove inflamed soft tissue from the luminal side of the posterior cushion and postero-medial wall. This surgical debulking removes inflamed and hypertrophied mucosa facilitating regrowth of healthy tissue, which is thought to both widen the lumen and permit more efficient dilatory action of the tensor veli palatini muscle. Several studies have looked at this procedure with success rates ranging from 36% to 92%. Tissue removal can be accomplished with either a laser or microdebrider and begins at the nasopharyngeal edge of the posterior cushion and extends up to the valve region. Within the valve region, resection of submucosal soft tissue is performed as necessary, but the mucosa is spared to prevent synechiae formation. An unusually prominent bulge of cartilage into the lumen can also be resected if necessary. It is important always to be oriented to the location of both the anterolateral wall and ICA and avoid damaging either structure.[18]

Although there is still a place for traditional tuboplasty, endoscopic balloon dilation of the cartilaginous ET has emerged over the past 5 years as the treatment of choice due to its high reported success rates ranging from 64% to 97%, and low risk profile and incidence complications of approximately 3%.[19] A significant advantage of balloon dilation is that it targets dilatory dysfunction at both the mucosal and muscular levels. Ilkka demonstrated histologic evidence that the balloon causes both shear and crush injury the epithelium, but spares the basal layer allowing for rapid healing. The balloon also crushes lymphocytes and lymphoid follicles within the submucosa leading to the formation of a fibrous scar. This combination significantly reduces the overall inflammatory burden and may provide lasting clinical improvement in both ET dilation and ventilation.[20] Muscle "tightness" or shortening has been shown to be due to an increase in tension and significantly limits range of motion. This increase in tension has been shown to be secondary to postural adaptation and/or scarring secondary to inflammatory process. The diameter of the ET ranges from 0.6 to 3.0 mm at the isthmus and 20.0 to 30.0 mm at the nasopharyngeal orifice. A fully dilated balloon usually has a diameter of 6 mm, causing significant stretch on peritubal musculature. The effect of this can be evaluated at looking at Hoffman reflexes (H-reflex) on electromyography. The H-reflex is a measurement of the muscle's level of excitability, and lower H-reflexes are associated with decreased excitability. Interestingly, H-reflexes have been found to be depressed with a precontraction stretch and the resultant decreased excitability of the muscle may allow the muscle to relax despite increased stimuli. This leads to a refractory period after contraction known as "autogenic inhibition," where muscle relaxes due to neuro-reflexive mechanisms, thus increasing muscle length.[21] Both of the proposed mechanisms of action of balloon dilation have been shown to take place primarily in the cartilaginous portion of the ET. This is important to note because not only do attempts to dilate the bony portion of the ET risk the ICA, which runs in close proximity to the osseous ET, but also limits the effectiveness of the balloon by restricting expansion and pressure on the cartilaginous ET. Multiple recent studies demonstrate that balloon dilation of the cartilaginous ET lumen is feasible, safe, and provides therapeutic benefit. Reported complications of balloon dilation of the ET include minor tears of the mucosal lumen, epistaxis, exacerbation of tinnitus, and subcutaneous emphysema, all of which resolved spontaneously.[19] Transnasal dilation of the cartilaginous ET is carried out using a 30 or 45° endoscope. Traditionally an angled guide catheter is used to introduce the 6 × 16-mm sinuplasty balloon into the nasopharyngeal orifice of the ET. It is useful to gently retract the posterior cushion medially to allow a view of the ET valve, providing guidance while advancing the balloon superiorly. The balloon catheter should be advanced until the 31-mm yellow mark is even with the medial edge of the anterior cushion or the catheter encounters resistance at the bony-cartilaginous isthmus. Inflation of the balloon has been described from either 10 or 12 atm for various time intervals; however, sustaining the dilation at 12 atm for 2 minutes is becoming the standard practice. Transnasal endoscopic ET dilation as performed by the authors is demonstrated in Video 1. There are several reports that deinflation followed by reinflation for 1 minute may be useful if there is a significant burden of disease. Extreme caution should be used when performing balloon dilation on patients who appear to have dehiscence of the carotid canal due to the possible although unlikely risk of inserting the balloon into the bony canal.[4]

In patients with patulous ET, myringotomy and tympanostomy tube placement has been shown to alleviate aural fullness and tympanic membrane excursions but is often ineffective for autophony.[5] Shim placement is a minimally invasive surgical option that can effectively relieve patulous symptoms while preserving ET function in most cases. Patients being considered for shim placement should undergo a preoperative CT scan to ensure that the ICA canal is not dehiscent. We perform shim placement under general anesthesia by using a polypropylene stylet obtained from a disposable 10-French catheter cut to size: 36 to 38 mm in female and 38 to 40 mm for male individuals. The distal centimeter of the catheter is then tapered to the diameter of the isthmus seen on CT reconstructions, usually this is approximately 2 mm. The catheter is then placed transnasally under 45° endoscopic guidance. The shim is first inserted into the end of a 70° curved guide catheter and then advanced with the remaining stylet. The shim is then slowly and atraumatically advanced into the lumen. Retraction of the posterior cushion straightens out the curvature of the ET, allowing for a view deep into the lumen until meeting resistance as it passes through the isthmus, steady firm pressure should then be placed at the end of the shim until it is seated within the lumen of the bony isthmus. The catheter is considered in good position once the distal end is flush with the free margin of the posterior cushion, just inside the anterior cushion. Most catheters remain lodged within the isthmus for years without any perception of its presence by the patient. The shim functions by lying within the concave defect in the valve, filling it sufficiently to restore competency to valve closure, surprisingly this usually occurs without occluding the ET. In the event of premature catheter extrusion, reconstruction of the patulous ET should be considered. Calcium hydroxyapatite paste augmentation of the ET luminal wall was initially reported as a standalone procedure, and resulted in complete or significant improvement in voice autophony 69% of the time; however, due to migration of the paste within the loose tissue planes of the anterolateral wall as well as a mild degree of absorption, symptom relief may be only temporary, thus requiring multiple injections. Because of these limitations, this procedure most often been regulated as a secondary procedure to augment deficient areas after soft tissue augmentation.[4] Soft tissue augmentation was initially described as an anterior lateral cartilage graft designed to reconstruct the deficient cartilaginous canal.[22] It is now this author's practice to make an incision along the anterior cushion and elevate the mucoperichondrium off the anterior wall of the ET, once the pocket is developed an autologous fat or fascial graft is placed followed by a tapered conchal cartilage graft in an attempt to both augment the anterior lateral wall as well as replicate the soft tissue consistency of a healthy ET. Transnasal endoscopic treatment of patulous ET as performed by the authors is shown in Video 2. If an element of patency to the ET remains, a vertical incision is then made in the posterior canal wall and the mucoperichondrium is elevated and a perichondrial graft is placed in the dissected space to augment the posterior wall and facilitate closure of the valve as demonstrated by the authors in Video 3. Due to the difficulty of placing effective sutures in this area, the remaining perichondrium is placed over the fat and cartilage in an underlay technique and covered with DuraSeal (Confluent Surgical Inc, Waltham, MA).

SUMMARY

Both dilatory and patulous dysfunction of the ET pose significant diagnostic and treatment challenges to the clinician. Recent advances in technology have led to a better understanding of the dynamic function of the ET, allowing for design and standardization of more effective diagnostic tests and validated symptom scores. This standardization allows us to effectively evaluate the various treatment options for ET disorders in an effort to determine when and in whom a specific option should be used. The treatment algorithm for ET disorders currently used by the authors is shown in **Fig. 1**. As

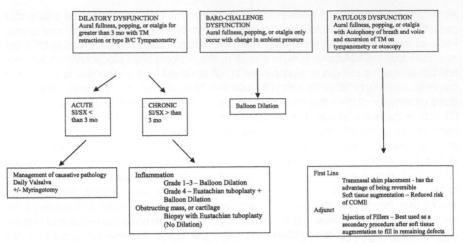

Fig. 1. Treatment algorithm for Eustachian tube disorders as recommended and practiced by the authors.

treatment algorithms become more refined and greater experience and long-term follow-up are obtained, it is likely that surgical intervention in the management of ET disorders will become standard of care, but until then extreme caution needs to be urged to avoid serious and unwanted complications.

SUPPLEMENTARY DATA

Supplementary data related to this article can be found online at http://dx.doi.org/10.1016/j.otc.2016.05.007.

REFERENCES

1. Silvola J, Kivekas I, Poe DS. Balloon dilation of the cartilaginous portion of the Eustachian tube. Otolaryngol Head Neck Surg 2014;151(1):125–30.
2. Ockermann T, Reineke U, Ebmeyer J, et al. Balloon dilatation eustachian tuboplasty: a clinical study. Laryngoscope 2010;120(7):1411–6.
3. Bluestone CD. Introduction. In: Bluestone, editor. Eustachian tube: structure, function, role in otitis media. Hamilton (ON): BC Decker Inc; 2005. p. 1–9.
4. Adil E, Poe DS. What is the full range of medical and surgical treatments available for patients with Eustachian tube dysfunction? Curr Opin Otolaryngol Head Neck Surg 2014;22(1):8–15.
5. Hussein A, Adams A, Turner J. Surgical management of patulous Eustachian tube: a systematic review. Laryngoscope 2015;125(9):2193–8.
6. Schilder AGM, Bhutta MF, Butler CC, et al. Eustachian tube dysfunction: consensus statement on definition, types, clinical presentation and diagnosis. Clin Otolaryngol 2015;40(5):407–11.
7. Seibert JW, Danner CJ. Eustachian tube function and the middle ear. Otolaryngol Clin North Am 2006;39(6):1221–35.
8. Browning GG, Gatehouse S. The prevalence of middle ear disease in the adult British population. Clin Otolaryngol 1992;17(4):317–21.
9. Poe DS, Pyykko I, Valtonen H, et al. Analysis of Eustachian tube function by video endoscopy. Am J Otol 2000;21(5):602–7.

10. Poe DS. Diagnosis and management of the patulous Eustachian tube. Otol Neurotol 2007;28(5):668–77.
11. McNicoll WD. Eustachian tube dysfunction in submariners and divers. Arch Otolaryngol 1982;108(5):279–83.
12. Llewellyn A, Norman G, Harden M, et al. Interventions for adult Eustachian tube dysfunction: a systematic review. Health Technol Assess 2014;18(46):1–180.
13. Doyle WJ, Swarts JD, Banks J, et al. Sensitivity and specificity of Eustachian tube function tests in adults. JAMA Otolaryngol Head Neck Surg 2013;139(7):719–27.
14. McCoul ED, Anand VK, Christos PJ. Validating the clinical assessment of eustachian tube dysfunction: the Eustachian Tube Dysfunction Questionnaire (ETDQ-7). Laryngoscope 2012;122(5):1137–41.
15. Van Roeyen S, Van de Heyning P, Van Rompaey P. Value and discriminative power of the seven-item Eustachian tube dysfunction questionnaire. Laryngoscope 2015;125(11):2553–6.
16. Gluth MB, McDonald DR, Weaver AL, et al. Management of Eustachian tube dysfunction with nasal steroid spray: a prospective, randomized, placebo-controlled trial. Arch Otolaryngol Head Neck Surg 2011;137(5):449–55.
17. Abdel-Aziz T, Schroder S, Lehmann M, et al. Computed tomography before balloon eustachian tuboplasty—a true necessity? Otol Neurotol 2014;35(4): 635–8.
18. Metson R, Pletcher SD, Poe DS. Microdebrider Eustachian tuboplasty: a preliminary report. Otolaryngol Head Neck Surg 2007;136(3):422–7.
19. Randrup T, Ovesen T. Balloon eustachian tuboplasty: a systematic review. Otolaryngol Head Neck Surg 2015;152(3):383–92.
20. Kivekäs I, Chao WC, Faquin W, et al. Histopathology of balloon-dilation Eustachian tuboplasty. Laryngoscope 2015;125(2):436–41.
21. Page P. Current concepts in muscle stretching for exercise and rehabilitation. Int J Sports Phys Ther 2012;7(1):109–19.
22. Doherty JK, Slattery WH 3rd. Autologous fat grafting for the refractory patulous Eustachian tube. Otolaryngol Head Neck Surg 2003;128(1):88–91.

Endoscopic Facial Nerve Surgery

Daniele Marchioni, MD[a], Davide Soloperto, MD[a], Alessia Rubini, MD[a],*,
João Flávio Nogueira, MD[b], Mohamed Badr-El-Dine, MD[c], Livio Presutti, MD[d]

KEYWORDS

- Facial nerve • Endoscopic approaches • Geniculate ganglion • Schwannomas
- Petrous bone fracture

KEY POINTS

- Endoscopic magnification of the tympanic cavity anatomy and good knowledge of middle ear structures allow a minimally invasive approach for the removal of disease.
- The transpromontorial approach allows eradication of lesions involving fundus of internal auditory canal and petrous apex, with limited extension to the intracochlear, intravestibular, and pericarotid regions.
- The suprageniculate approach allows eradication of pathologic conditions involving the triangular area between geniculate ganglion inferiorly, middle cranial fossa dura superiorly, and labyrinthic bloc posteriorly.
- Endoscopic transcanal facial nerve decompression is applicable in cases of posttraumatic facial palsy, in particular, when there is an involvement of the geniculate ganglion region.
- The endoscopic approach allows a complete exposure of the facial nerve course, from the labyrinthic tract to the second genu, with low morbidity.

INTRODUCTION

The dissemination of endoscopic ear surgery in the otological community in the last decade expanded the use of the external auditory canal (EAC) as a natural surgical corridor to access diseases located in the tympanic cavity.[1] Several investigators have described the use of exclusive endoscopic transcanal approaches to tympanic cavity cholesteatomas.[2]

These approaches allowed also an improvement of the tympanic cavity anatomic knowledge, especially over the last 5 years. In fact, several studies in

The authors have nothing to disclose.
[a] Otolaryngology Department, University Hospital of Verona, Borgo Trento Piazza Aristide Stefani Aristide Stefani 1, Verona 37100, Italy; [b] Sinus and Oto Centro–Hospital Geral de Fortaleza, Rua Dr. José Furtado, 1480, Fortaleza 60822-300, Brazil; [c] Otolaryngology Department, University Hospital of Alexandria, 36 Rouschdy Street #6, Rouschdy, Alexandria, Egypt; [d] Otolaryngology Department, University Hospital of Modena, Via del Pozzo 71, Modena 41100, Italy
* Corresponding author.
E-mail address: rubinialessia@gmail.com

Otolaryngol Clin N Am 49 (2016) 1173–1187
http://dx.doi.org/10.1016/j.otc.2016.05.006
0030-6665/16/$ – see front matter © 2016 Elsevier Inc. All rights reserved.
oto.theclinics.com

literature were focused on the endoscopic anatomy of the retrotympanum and epitympanum.[3,4]

Recently, the endoscopic anatomy from the EAC to the internal auditory canal (IAC) was described in detail, and this allowed also the identification of the facial nerve pathway from the second genu until the geniculate ganglion (GG), and from the GG to the intralabyrinthine segment of the facial nerve into the IAC.[5]

Moreover, using the EAC as a natural surgical corridor, the investigators described the possibility of reaching the tympanic segment of the facial nerve, studying the anatomic conformation and its relationships with the surrounding anatomic structures.[3]

The continued progress of the facial nerve endoscopic anatomy knowledge permitted an advancement in surgery, performing facial nerve transcanal exclusive endoscopic surgery for the treatment of facial nerve diseases located on its tympanic portion, GG, and suprageniculate fossa.[6,7]

ANATOMICAL CONSIDERATIONS

From an endoscopic point of view, it is possible to consider the tympanic facial nerve into 2 portions regarding the orientation to the cochleariform process (CP): precochleariform and postcochleariform segments.[3]

Precochleariform Segment of Tympanic Portion of Facial Nerve

Precochleariform segment is the portion of the tympanic facial nerve lying superiorly and anteriorly to the posterior bony limit of the CP.

This segment of the facial nerve is composed by the GG and the greater petrosal nerve (GPN). It is necessary to remove the malleus head to obtain good visualization of the precochleariform segment and the GG area.

The precochleariform segment has a parallel orientation with respect to semicanal of tensor tendon of the malleus, lying superiorly to this semicanal. Microscopic access to the anterior epitympanum should be made by a mastoidectomy, posterior atticotomy, and removal of the incus and head of the malleus.

On the other hand, after ossicular chain removal, which can be considered mandatory, the GG can be easily accessed using an exclusive endoscopic transcanal route, with the advantages of sparing mastoid tissues and avoiding more extended approaches.

Therefore, endoscopy guarantees true advantages compared with microscopy in terms of surgical maneuvering and access of extreme anterior segment of the tympanic facial nerve toward the GG (**Fig. 1**A).

Geniculate Ganglion

The CP represents an excellent landmark to identify the GG, which is located just medially and superiorly to the CP.

GG is in the floor of the anterior epitympanic space and has a horizontal orientation parallel to the semicanal of the tensor tendon of the malleus (**Fig. 1**B).

In 66.7% of cases, the GG is covered by the bone of the anterior epitympanic space cells, so in these cases the cells of the anterior epitympanic space just anteriorly and superiorly to the CP should be removed in order to expose the GG.

From literature, in 33.3% of cases a partial dehiscence of the ganglion in the anterior epitympanic space cells was found.[3]

Another anatomic landmark for GG is the transverse crest, which is a bony ridge extending inferiorly from the tegmen tympani of the anterior epitympanic space, just anterior to the CP, also known as the "COG" (**Fig. 1**B).[8,9]

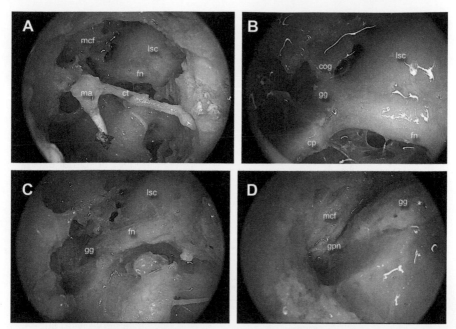

Fig. 1. Cadaveric dissection left ear. (*A*) The incus and the head of the malleus was removed, providing a wide access to the facial nerve. (*B*) Endoscopic closer view on the GG; this anatomic structure is located between the CP and the transversal crest (cog). (*C*) The malleus was removed and GG was exposed removing the epitympanic cells. (*D*) The endoscopic magnification of the relationship of the GG, the GPN, and the dura of the middle fossa. cp, cochleariform process; ct, corda tympani; fn, facial nerve; gg, geniculate ganglion; gpn, greater petrosal nerve; lsc, lateral semicircular canal; ma, malleus; mcf, middle cranial fossa.

The transverse crest is not always clearly described in the literature, and a frequent variability of this structure is noted. It has different conformations and relationships to the GG, tensor fold, and supratubal recess. From recent work, it can be considered different conformation of the COG.

In the authors' series, the COG is a complete bony crest in 58.3% of cases, having a transverse inclination attaching anteriorly and superiorly to the most anterior portion of the tegmen tympani. In these cases, the transverse crest "indicates" posteriorly and inferiorly the CP, and it is a landmark for the GG during transcanal endoscopic approach. On the other hand, in 41.7% of cases, an incomplete or rudimental transverse crest was found, in close relationship to the tegmen of the anterior epitympanic space. When incomplete or rudimental, the transverse crest could not be considered a true landmark for the GG, either because it does not clearly indicate the ganglion or because it lies significantly anteriorly and laterally to the nerve.[3]

The location of the GG is shown by these 2 anatomic structures. The GG is found lying just superiorly and anteriorly with respect to the CP, whereas the COG descends from the tegmen like a finger, indicating the location of the ganglion (**Fig. 2**).

Greater Petrosal Nerve

Endoscopic access to the GPN is obtained by removing the head of the malleus in order to reach good access to the anterior bony wall of the anterior epitympanic space. It is necessary to remove the transverse crest and the supratubal recess (when present),

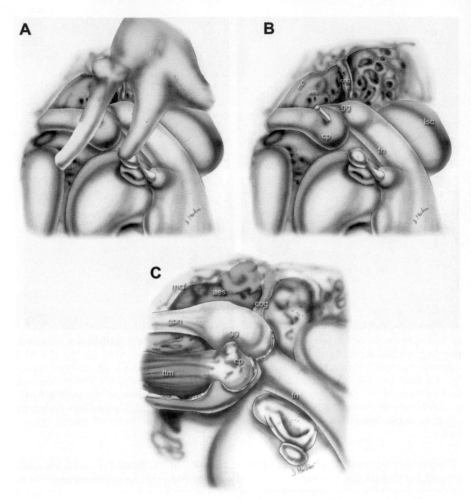

Fig. 2. Left ear: schematic drawing representing the anatomy of the precochleariform area and landmarks used during the transcanal endoscopic approach. (*A*) Tympanic cavity after tympanomeatal flap elevation; note that the ossicular chain covers the precochleariform area of the facial nerve. (*B*) Anatomy of the tympanic segment of the facial nerve after ossicular chain removal; the traditional landmarks for GG localization are present; the cog descends from the tegmen and, like a finger, indicates the GG area. The CP is located just under and posteriorly with respect to the GG. (*C*) Close-up view of the precochleariform area; the tensor tendon bony canal was removed to uncover the homonymous muscle. Note the close relationship between the GG and the CP; the GPN is evident anteriorly with respect to the GG. It runs parallel to the tensor tendon canal, and the MCF descends anteriorly, reaching the GPN. aes, anterior epitympanic space; ttm, muscle of the tensor tendon of the malleus.

anteriorly to the GG, in order to expose the GPN, following the anterior orientation of the facial nerve (**Fig. 1**C).[3]

In 40% of cases, a dehiscence of the middle cranial fossa (MCF) dura is observed at the anterior epitympanic space, and the dura of the MCF is in a close relationship with both, the GG and the GPN (**Fig. 1**D).

On the contrary, in 60% of cases, it is necessary to drill in order to find the dura of the MCF.[5]

Postcochleariform Segment of Tympanic Portion of Facial Nerve

The postcochleariform segment is the portion of the tympanic facial nerve lying posteriorly to the posterior bony limit of the CP. This segment represents the floor of the posterior epitympanic space.[3]

In 75% of cases, the postcochleariform segment has a slightly oblique orientation to the semicanal of the tensor tendon of the malleus, descending above the oval window and the stapes from the CP anteriorly to the second genu.

In 25% of cases, this segment has a parallel orientation to the semicanal of the tensor tendon of the malleus. The postcochleariform segment is parallel with respect to the lateral semicircular canal. That landmark is important in order to reach the aditus ad antrum endoscopically.

In the most posterior portion, in the transition zone between the tympanic and mastoid segment, the facial nerve becomes transcanally inaccessible by microscope, whereby a mastoidectomy is required to reach this area.

On the other hand, the transcanal endoscopic approach allows a direct route to the postcochleariform segment of the facial nerve after incus and head of the malleus removal, sparing mastoid tissues and wide external incisions. The only portion of facial nerve that does not require ossicular chain removal to be exposed is the most posterior, in close relationship with the second genu and the pyramidal eminence.[3]

Intralabyrinthine portion of facial nerve

The intralabyrinthine portion of facial nerve runs from the GG to the IAC anteriorly to posteriorly, and to the fundus of the IAC, laterally to medially.[10]

The medial turn of the cochlea represents an important landmark for the intralabyrinthine facial nerve, because this segment of the nerve runs just superiorly to the cochlea from the GG superiorly and anteriorly, and the intrameatal facial nerve inferiorly and posteriorly (**Fig. 3**C).

The intralabyrinthine tract of the facial nerve from the IAC to the GG could be identified by drilling an anatomic triangle between the GG superiorly, the basal turn of the cochlea anteriorly, and the spherical recess IAC posteroinferiorly.

The intralabyrinthine facial nerve is covered by a compact bony wall, and the dissection of this component of the facial nerve is quite difficult and could be exposed and visualized by drilling between the GG and the cochlea anteriorly, and the medial wall of the vestibule, and the IAC posteriorly. Although the intralabyrinthine facial nerve was covered by a compact bony wall, it is extremely fragile, and at this point, the facial nerve has its smallest diameter so it could be easily damaged.[5]

TRANSCANAL ENDOSCOPIC APPROACHES TO THE FACIAL NERVE

The initial experiences of the transcanal endoscopic approaches to the facial nerve started with cadaveric dissections and, after codification of different approaches based on anatomy, clinical and surgical experiences were made, using endoscopic techniques for different pathologic conditions, such as traumatic, inflammatory, and neoplastic problems.[5,6,10]

Current endoscopic approaches to the facial nerve described in literature are as follows:

- The endoscopic transcanal transpromontorial approach[6,11]
- The endoscopic transcanal suprageniculate approach[6,7]
- The endoscopic transcanal facial nerve decompression[5]

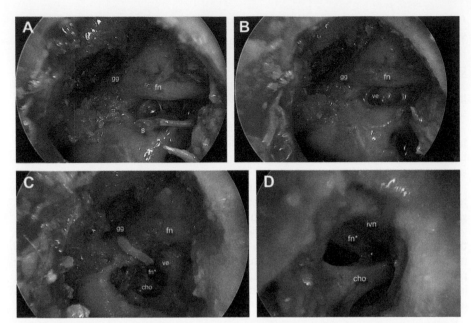

Fig. 3. Cadaveric dissection left ear. (*A*) The GG was exposed and the ossicular chain was removed. (*B*) The stapes was removed entering in the vestibule. (*C*) The cochlea is opened, and the bony wall between the cochlea and the vestibule was removed entering into the IAC exposing the cochlear nerve. The labyrinthine segment of the facial nerve runs from the GG just upper the cochlea to the fundus of the IAC (*yellow line*). (*D*) Closer endoscopic view of the fundus of the IAC. cho, cochlea; fn*, facial nerve into the IAC; ivn, inferior vestibular nerve; s, stapes; ve, vestibule.

The aim of this article is to describe the authors' experience with the transcanal endoscopic approach to the diseases involving the facial nerve, describing assumptions, indications, and procedures.

Endoscopic Transcanal Transpromontorial Approach

Indications[6,11]

- Facial nerve schwannomas involving the labyrinthic and tympanic tract of the facial nerve, with or without facial palsy;
- Symptomatic or growing cochlear schwannomas, with or without extension to the fundus of the IAC;
- Symptomatic or growing acoustic neuromas, with exclusive extension of the fundus of the IAC;
- Mesotympanic cholesteatomas, with medial extension to the inner ear.
- Symptomatic residual tumors located at the fundus of the IAC.

Advantages

- Direct exposure of the fundus of the IAC, with lower morbidity when compared with traditional surgery.

Disadvantages

- Hearing loss is expected, because of the drilling of the cochlea to reach the IAC, so a preoperative hearing status evaluation is mandatory for the correct indication

With this surgical approach, the fundus of the IAC is reached by passing through the promontory, using the EAC as a door for access, and disease must be located in the vestibule, cochlea, and/or IAC.[11]

Surgical steps
A circumferential incision is made on the EAC, 2 cm from the tympanic membrane, and a wide tympanomeatal flap is realized by skin degloving. The entire eardrum with the meatal skin flap of the EAC is removed. A diamond burr is used to perform a wide meatoplasty, and the bony annulus is drilled circumferentially until the hypotympanum, retrotympanum, and protympanum are exposed endoscopically so as to obtain optimal surgical space and control of the whole medial wall of the tympanic cavity. The scutum is removed to uncover the incudomalleolar joint. The incus is removed, and the tensor tendon is cut, removing the malleus. Using a hook, the stapes is removed to expose the vestibule (**Fig. 3**A, B). The spherical recess, representing the cribrose area where the inferior vestibular nerve is attached and a landmark for the IAC, is detected endoscopically in the saccular fossa. When the disease involves the vestibule without IAC extension, the oval window opening is enlarged inferiorly on the promontory using a microcurette, allowing direct access to the medial wall of the vestibule, and the disease from the depth of the vestibule is carefully removed endoscopically. This latter surgical maneuver is performed carefully to avoid trauma to the spherical recess and consequent cerebrospinal fluid (CSF) leakage. When the disease is located in the cochlea with or without IAC involvement, a more anterior transcochlear approach could be performed. The round window membrane is detected, and the tegmen of the round window is removed. Using a Piezosurgery device (Mectron, Carasco/Genova, Italy), the promontory is completely removed to gain access to the cochlea. During this procedure, the basal, middle, and upper turns of the cochlea are progressively identified. The upper portion of the medial turn of the cochlea is identified and used as a landmark for location of the labyrinthine tract of the facial nerve (see **Fig. 3**C). Dissection of the cochlea is performed progressively until the helicotrema is identified. Dissection of the cochlea is performed progressively, detecting the fundus of the IAC and allowing the cochlear nerve entrance to be seen (**Fig. 3**C, D). When the disease is located in the cochlea, a gentle dissection of the tumor is performed, trying to avoid CSF leakage. When the tumor is located in the IAC, the fundus of the IAC is carefully opened through the cochlea just below the vestibule and the spherical recess, exposing the lesion in the IAC. During this surgical maneuver, an outflow of CSF occurs. By gently maneuvering the tumor mass, the facial nerve is detected endoscopically; then, the tumor mass is dissected from the IAC and from the facial nerve, paying careful attention not to damage the nerve. Afterward, a final inspection of the surgical cavity and the IAC is made to confirm complete removal of the mass. Closure of the IAC is performed with abdominal fat, packing the promontorial defect and closing the communication between the inner and middle ear. Fibrin glue is used to secure the closure of the promontorial defect. Depending on the extent of the disease and the extent of tissue extirpation, either repositioning of the tympanic membrane and ear canal skin with a tragal graft underlay or a cul-de-sac closure of the skin of the EAC is performed.

Endoscopic Transcanal Suprageniculate Approach

Indications (**Fig. 4**)[6,7]
- Abnormalities involving the tympanic tract of the facial nerve, especially located between the GG and the second genu of the facial nerve, with an infralabyrinthic extension, into the suprageniculate triangle (facial nerve hemangiomas, schwannomas, cholesteatomas) (**Figs. 5** and **6**).

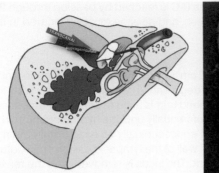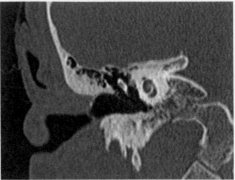

Fig. 4. The transcanal endoscopic suprageniculate approach: on the left, the surgical route from the EAC to the suprageniculate fossa (*arrow*); on the right, the CT scan in coronal view shows the working area and the bony removal (*yellow area*) between the MCF and the facial nerve into the petrous apex over the cochlea, which may be performed with this approach.

Advantages
- Direct and mini-invasive exposure of the tympanic tract of the facial nerve, especially for the most anterior portion, with particular attention to the CP area.
- Lower morbidity with respect to traditional surgery, avoiding temporal lobe traction and postoperative CSF leak.

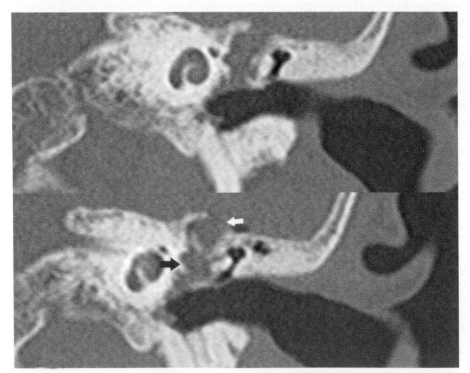

Fig. 5. CT scan: coronal view showing a tympanic cavity cholesteatoma involving the suprageniculate fossa between the GG (*black arrow*) and the MCF (*white arrow*). The transcanal endoscopic suprageniculate approach may be used as a surgical route in this case.

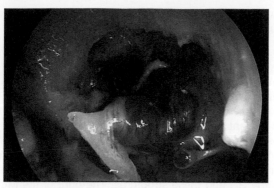

Fig. 6. Transcanal endoscopic suprageniculate approach: a facial nerve hemangioma is exposed endoscopically through the EAC.

- Hearing function preservation.

Disadvantages

- Ossicular chain disarticulation (incus and malleus head removal), with necessity of ossiculoplasty and a variable postoperative conductive hearing loss.
- When a dural repair is associated, a combined microscopic approach is necessary.

This approach through the EAC is realized when the disease is located between the GG and the second portion of the facial nerve inferiorly, the MCF lying superiorly, and the labyrinthine bloc posteriorly. Working above the cochlea and labyrinth (**Fig. 7**),

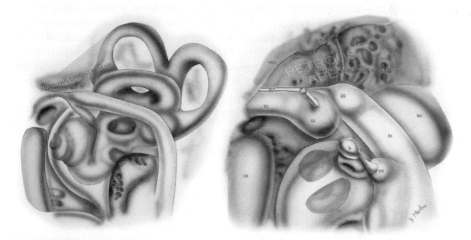

Fig. 7. Left ear. The transcanal endoscopic suprageniculate approach: on the left, the transcanal anatomy of the medial wall of the tympanic cavity related to the working area of the transcanal suprageniculate approach (*orange area*). On the right, the endoscopic transcanal anatomic landmarks in this approach; the orange area indicates the bony area between the MCF superiorly, the facial nerve and GG inferiorly, and the labyrinthine block posteriorly, which may be removed to reach the petrous apex endoscopically. ca, carotid artery; et, Eustachian tube; pe, pyramidal eminence; pes, posterior epitympanic space; ttc, tensor tendon canal.

sensorineural hearing function is preserved. An ossiculoplasty is usually required at the end of the surgery, due to the necessity of malleus and incus disarticulation in order to correctly expose the second tract of the facial nerve.[6]

Surgical steps

A wide tympanomeatal flap is created from 11 o'clock to 6 o'clock to expose the tympanic cavity; the flap is then transposed inferiorly and detached from the handle of the malleus to obtain good exposure of the medial wall of the tympanic cavity. When the ossicular chain is present and intact, removal of the incus and head of the malleus is required to expose the entire second portion of the facial nerve, from the second genu to the GG and the GPN area. The COG and the CP are identified endoscopically and used as an anatomic landmark for the GG area owing to the close anatomic relationship between the GG and these structures. The dura of the MCF is exposed by removing bone from the tegmen of the anterior epitympanum and represented the upper surgical limit. The lateral semicircular canal is also detected endoscopically, posteriorly, and superiorly, with respect to the second genu of the facial nerve, representing the posterior limit of the surgical dissection. The COG is gently removed using a microcurette, increasing the exposure of the GG area, and when required, the GPN is also exposed just anteriorly to the GG. Based on the extent of the disease, a diamond burr or a Piezosurgery device (Mectron) is used to remove the bone between the MCF superiorly, the labyrinthine bloc posteriorly, and the facial nerve inferiorly, reaching the pathologic tissue in this area. After disease removal, a fragment of temporal muscle is used to obliterate the cavity created; an ossicular chain reconstruction is performed at the same time as the surgery, and the tympanomeatal flap is replaced.

Postoperative care and follow-up

A brain computed tomographic (CT) scan on the first postoperative day or several hours after the operation is performed to rule out complications. Intravenous antibiotic therapy (third-generation cephalosporin) is administered for 48 hours after surgery.

The facial nerve function (House-Brackmann scale) is evaluated immediately after surgery and during the follow-up time. An otoendoscopic examination is performed postoperatively after 1 month. Other otoendoscopic examinations with audiologic examinations are performed at 4, 6, and 12 months after surgery.

Endoscopic Transcanal Facial Nerve Decompression

Indications[5]
- Posttraumatic facial nerve palsy, with perigeniculate region involvement (as in **Fig. 8**).

Advantages
- Direct and mini-invasive exposure of the tympanic tract of the facial nerve, in particular, exposure of the tympanic tract of the GG and GPN;
- Lower morbidity when compared with traditional surgery, avoiding temporal lobe traction or postoperative CSF leak.

Disadvantages
- Ossicular chain disarticulation (incus and malleus head removal), with necessity of ossiculoplasty and a variable postoperative conductive hearing loss;
- When a dural repair is associated, a combined microscopic approach is necessary.

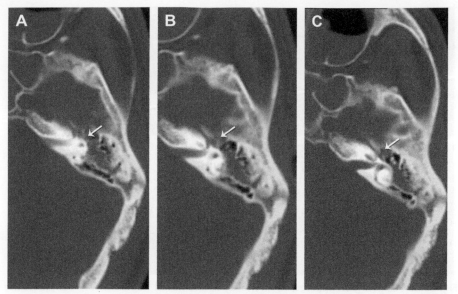

Fig. 8. (*A–C*) CT scan in axial view. Note the fracture of the temporal bone involving the GG area (*arrow*) anteriorly with respect to the ossicular chain.

The transcanal endoscopic decompression of the tympanic segment of the facial nerve allows a good exposure of the second genu and of the most anterior portion of the nerve, in particular, the region lying anterior to the CP, in close proximity to the GG, the anterior epitympanum and the supratubal recess are correctly showed, without a transmastoid posterior atticotomy.

Surgical steps
Using the 0° endoscopic view, an incision of the EAC is performed with a round knife from 11 o'clock to 6 o'clock. A tympanomeatal flap is endoscopically elevated, anteriorly and inferiorly based; the eardrum is gently detached from the malleus, cutting the adhesion located in the umbus between the eardrum and the handle of the malleus. The tympano-meatal flap is gently pulled inferiorly in order to uncover the whole scutum and the rim of the fracture involving the pregeniculate area (as in **Fig. 9**A). The scutum is partially drilled, allowing adequate access to the anterior epitympanum. The bony fragments from the fracture involving the pregeniculate area and the anterior epitympanum are carefully removed, maintaining the integrity of the ossicular chain (**Fig. 9**B). The CP and the COG are detected endoscopically, representing important landmarks for the location of the GG (**Fig. 9**C). Then, the anterior wall of the scutum is extensively removed. In this way, a better endoscopic view of the precochleariform area is obtained. A bony fragment compressing the GPN is removed and the nerve detected (**Fig. 9**D).

In order to generate more surgical control in the entire precochleariform area, the malleus is disarticulated from the incus, and then gently pulled down, leaving it attached to the tensor tympani tendon (**Fig. 10**A). After this procedure, the tympanic segment of the facial nerve with the GG area is visible endoscopically, giving a wide working area (**Fig. 10**B, C). The decompression of the whole tympanic segment is easily performed under endoscopic view. The fracture on the GG is detected, and the bony fragments pressing on the GG are carefully removed using a small dissector. The decompression of the GG is performed until the GPN is reached. After this proce-dure, a Gelfoam soaked with corticosteroid solution is placed in the surgical field,

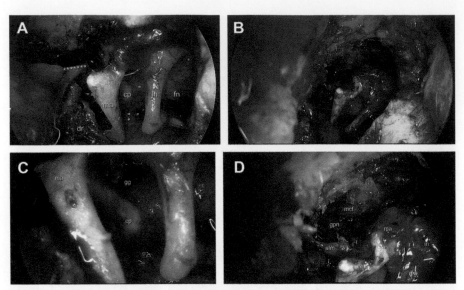

Fig. 9. Left ear. Surgical approach. (*A*) After tympanomeatal flap elevation, the rim of the fracture is seen endoscopically, running from the anterior wall of the EAC to the preco-chleariform area. (*B*) Decompression of the precochleariform area is performed: the scutum with bony fragments from the fracture involving the precochleariform area is removed to reveal the anterior epitympanic space, maintaining the integrity of the ossicular chain. (*C*) Through the isthmus, the GG area and its relationship with the CP are detected endoscopically. (*D*) The precochleariform area, where the fracture is located, is recognized endoscopically, the GPN with its relationship to the MCF is also evident; the malleus partially covers the GG. alm, anterior ligament of the malleus; dr, eardrum; in, incus; ma, malleus.

close to the facial nerve, and the malleus is gently repositioned on the incus, restoring the integrity of the ossicular chain (**Fig. 10**D). A cartilage graft, harvested from the tragus, is used to reconstruct the tegmen defect. The tympanomeatal flap is repositioned, and the EAC is filled with Gelfoam.

Postoperative care and follow-up

During the hospital stay, intravenous corticosteroids and antibiotics (third-generation cephalosporin) are administered, followed by antibiotic and corticosteroid oral therapy at discharge.

The facial nerve function (HB scale) is evaluated immediately after surgery and during the follow-up time. An otoendoscopic evaluation is performed postoperatively after 1 month. Other otoendoscopic examinations with audiologic examinations are performed at 4, 6, and 12 months from surgery.

DISCUSSION

The adoption of middle ear endoscopic surgery is gradually spreading through the otological community, and this is mainly because endoscopes with various degrees of angulation allow the surgeon to "see around corners" to visualize hidden spaces, even the smallest and least accessible, such as the retrotympanum or anterior epitympanum, also providing a magnification effect when close to objects. Although at the initial attempts, the endoscope was used with only an explorative aim and operations were mainly performed using microscopic aid, their exclusive use in ear surgery is gradually diffusing.

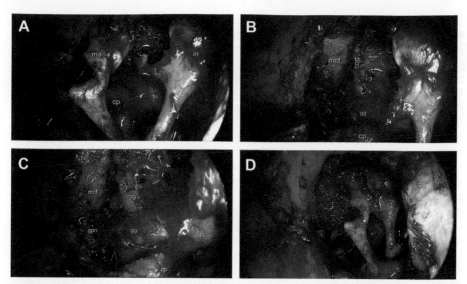

Fig. 10. Left ear. (*A*) In order to obtain a wide view of the entire precochleariform area, the malleus is disarticulated from the incus and pulled down maintaining its adhesion with the tensor tendon medially and the anterior ligament anteriorly. (*B*) The precochleariform area is completely visible endoscopically, and all the landmarks for facial nerve recognition are seen. (*C*) Endoscopic magnification after nerve decompression of the precochleariform area. The GG is located just superiorly and anteriorly with respect to the CP. The cog descends from the tegmen, and, like a finger, indicates where the GG is located. The GPN runs anteriorly with respect to the GG, and along the course of the nerve, it joins with the MCF. (*D*) The malleus is repositioned on the incus, and the anterior epitympanum is filled with Gelfoam soaked with corticosteroid solution.

This use of the endoscope introduced new anatomic and surgical concepts.[12,13] Dealing with surgical approaches to the facial nerve, classical transcanal microscopic procedures are well known, and enable visualization of most of the tympanic segment of the facial nerve apart from regions such as those at its extreme anterior part, and extending toward the GG[6]: in these cases, access to the anterior epitympanum should be made by a mastoidectomy and posterior atticotomy, and, of course, with removal of the incus and head of the malleus.[8,9]

On the other hand, the GG can be easily and quickly accessed by an exclusive endoscopic transcanal approach, hence sparing mastoid tissues and avoiding more extensive approaches. This finding could have quite important clinical relevance, because, for example, the most common segment involved in posttraumatic facial nerve palsy is considered to be the perigeniculate region.[8,9] In the case of a finding consistent with a fracture involving that region, traditional approaches to the GG and intralabyrinthine tract of the facial nerve for trauma would be by a MCF approach, or, in the case of hearing loss after trauma, also by a translabyrinthine approach.

For abnormalities with fundus of the IAC and labyrinthic tract of the facial nerve involvement, traditional microscopic surgery usually consists of open approaches, with hard dissection and very extensive bone removal, in order to expose these anatomic regions. From several experiences, based on cadaveric dissections and recent clinical advances, the facial nerve can be visualized quite easily by endoscopic techniques, using a transcanal exclusive surgery, even in the most anterior, posterior, or medial extension. This approach allows complete control of the facial nerve in its tympanic tract, GG, GPN, and labyrinthic tract. The pathologic tissue can be removed safely, and further bone removal is performed, based on the pathologic condition. The advantages are represented by a mini-invasive surgery, with a lower morbidity if compared with microscopic surgery, for example, MCF approach or translabyrinthic approach, in fact the possibility of complete facial nerve exposure, without extensive bone drilling typical of microscopic approaches, making this surgery very useful in all these diseases. Of course, the transcanal endoscopic approach may have some limitations. First of all, adequate dimensions of the external ear canal are mandatory in performing the complex endoscopic surgical maneuver. In fact, all the procedures are performed by only one hand, and this could be difficult for an inexperienced surgeon. In particular, one should be careful of the stapes during procedures around the postcochleariform segment of facial nerve, and the use of small burrs may represent a good option for this. Moreover, as is also true in all the middle ear endoscopic procedures, excessive intraoperative bleeding may force the surgeon to switch to a microscopic approach, so that it is possible to hold with the second hand a suction device during the operation. The use of endoscopic approaches requires, for complete visualization of the facial nerve, incus disarticulation and removal, so in these cases the endoscope does not give advantages in terms of ossicular chain preservation compared with microscopic techniques: any way the incus can be replaced at the end of the operation or an ossiculoplasty can be performed instead. Moreover, in several cases, a microscopic procedure is required to manage the dural defect with CSF leakage, because this could be a difficult surgical step if performed endoscopically.

SUMMARY

The tympanic facial nerve can be thoroughly visualized using an exclusive endoscopic transcanal approach, even in poorly accessible regions such as the second genu and GG, avoiding mastoidectomy, bony demolition, and meningeal or cerebral lobe tractions. However, several studies are necessary to standardize the technique, and future widespread application of this kind of approach will depend on the development of technology and surgical and anatomic refinements.

REFERENCES

1. Kozin ED, Gulati S, Kaplan AB, et al. Systematic review of outcomes following observational and operative endoscopic middle ear surgery. Laryngoscope 2015;125(5):1205–14.
2. Presutti L, Gioacchini FM, Alicandri-Ciufelli M, et al. Results of endoscopic middle ear surgery for cholesteatoma treatment: a systematic review. Acta Otorhinolaryngol Ital 2014;34(3):153–7.
3. Marchioni D, Alicandri-Ciufelli M, Piccinini A, et al. Surgical anatomy of transcanal endoscopic approach to the tympanic facial nerve. Laryngoscope 2011;121(7): 1565–73.
4. Marchioni D, Molteni G, Presutti L. Endoscopic anatomy of the middle ear. Indian J Otolaryngol Head Neck Surg 2011;63(2):101–13.
5. Marchioni D, Alicandri-Ciufelli M, Mattioli F, et al. From external to internal auditory canal: surgical anatomy by an exclusive endoscopic approach. Eur Arch Otorhinolaryngol 2013;270(4):1267–75.
6. Marchioni D, Alicandri-Ciufelli M, Rubini A, et al. Endoscopic transcanal corridors to the lateral skull base: initial experiences. Laryngoscope 2016;125(Suppl 5): S1–13.

7. Marchioni D, Soloperto D, Genovese E, et al. Facial nerve hemangioma of the geniculate ganglion: an endoscopic surgical approach. Auris Nasus Larynx 2014;41(6):576–8.
8. Jenkins HA, Ator GA. Traumatic facial paralysis. In: Brackmann DE, Shelton C, Arriaga MA, editors. Otologic surgery. 2nd edition. Philadelphia: Saunders; 2001. p. 329. Chapter 30.
9. Sanna M, Sunose H, Mancini F, et al. Anatomy of temporal bone. In: Middle ear and mastoid microsurgery. Stuttgart (Germany): Georg Thieme Verlag; 2003. Chapter 1.
10. Presutti L, Alicandri-Ciufelli M, Rubini A, et al. Combined lateral microscopic/endoscopic approaches to petrous apex lesions: pilot clinical experiences. Ann Otol Rhinol Laryngol 2014;123(8):550–9.
11. Presutti L, Alicandri-Ciufelli M, Cigarini E, et al. Cochlear schwannoma removed through the external auditory canal by a transcanal exclusive endoscopic technique. Laryngoscope 2013;123(11):2862–7.
12. Marchioni D, Alicandri-Ciufelli M, Piccinini A, et al. Inferior retrotympanum revisited: an endoscopic anatomic study. Laryngoscope 2010;120(9):1880–6.
13. Tarabichi M. Endoscopic management of limited attic cholesteatoma. Laryngoscope 2004;114(7):1157–62.

Endoscopic-Assisted Repair of Superior Canal Dehiscence

Yew Song Cheng, BM BCh[a,b], Elliott D. Kozin, MD[a,b], Daniel J. Lee, MD[a,b],*

KEYWORDS

- Endoscopic ear surgery • Superior canal dehiscence
- Superior canal dehiscence syndrome • Lateral skull base • Middle fossa craniotomy
- Endoscope • Otology

KEY POINTS

- Middle fossa craniotomy (MFC) and transmastoid approaches are the most common surgical techniques to repair superior canal dehiscence (SCD). The advantage of the MFC approach is direct visualization and surgical access to the SCD without the need for drilling the skull base in most cases.
- Endoscopes provide a superior view (compared with binocular microscopy) of arcuate eminence defects using a MFC approach, especially medial dehiscences that are found along the downsloping tegmen.
- Improved visualization of arcuate eminence defect using the endoscope is achieved with a minimally invasive skin, soft tissue and craniotomy approach, with reduced temporal lobe retraction, and avoidance of drilling overlying bony ridges that obscure the line of sight.
- Endoscopes provide superior transillumination of the skull base and localization of blue-lined superior canals, which is important when repairing symptomatic "near dehiscence" SCD.
- Massachusetts Eye and Ear radiologic classification of SCD and surrounding skull base topography is helpful in preoperative planning and can anticipate the need for an endoscopic-guided repair.

INTRODUCTION

First characterized by Minor and colleagues[1] in 1998, superior canal dehiscence (SCD) is a bony defect of the superior canal that is associated with vestibular and/or auditory dysfunction. Classic symptoms associated with SCD syndrome (SCDS) include aural

Disclosures: None.
Conflict of Interest: None.
[a] Department of Otolaryngology, Massachusetts Eye and Ear Infirmary, 243 Charles Street, Boston, MA 02114, USA; [b] Department of Otology and Laryngology, Harvard Medical School, 25 Shattuck Street, Boston, MA 02115, USA
* Corresponding author. Massachusetts Eye and Ear Infirmary, 243 Charles Street, Boston, MA 02114.
E-mail address: Daniel_Lee@MEEi.harvard.edu

fullness, pulsating tinnitus, autophony, and conductive hyperacusis (hearing one's own voice, footsteps, and/or eye movements in the affected ear) and dizziness or vertigo evoked by loud sounds (Tullio phenomenon) or Valsalva maneuver (Hennebert sign).[2] Symptoms can vary widely among patients with SCDS, and not all patients with these defects have symptoms.

The concept of a pathologic mobile "third window" of the inner ear (the oval and round windows being the first two) is widely accepted as the explanation for SCDS pathophysiology.[3–6] Based on this concept, it is hypothesized that a third window allows for transmission of fluid pressure between the intralabyrinthine space and the cranial vault.[4,7–10] With this alternative path of low impedance, acoustic flow entering from the oval window is shunted toward the dehiscence causing hearing loss and deflection of the superior canal cupula away from the ampulla (ampullofugal) resulting in the stimulation of the affected superior canal.[3] Conversely, straining or Valsalva against closed glottis can lead to labyrinthine fluid flow away from the dehiscence and toward the ampulla (ampullopetal) resulting in inhibition of the superior canal ampulla.[11] Dizziness and vertigo can arise from either condition. Hypersensitivity to sounds and vibrations conducted through the body is a common feature of SCDS and is thought to be part of the third window phenomenon, but the underlying mechanism is still a subject of ongoing research.

Conservative management is adequate for most patients with SCDS, but for patients with severe symptoms, surgical repair is a feasible option.[12,13] Microscopic-assisted middle fossa craniotomy (MFC) is a widely used technique to repair SCDs because it is well-established and safe.[14,15] Alternatively, some surgeons favor a less invasive transmastoid approach to either directly repair the dehiscence (through a tegmen defect created from the mastoid area)[16–20] or indirectly isolating the dehiscence (by creating labyrinthotomies on either side of the SCD and then plugging the canal).[21–23] At the Massachusetts Eye and Ear Infirmary (MEEI) we believe that the transmastoid approach is ideal for SCDs associated with the superior petrosal sinus (**Fig. 1E**)[24] and revision cases, where the MFC approach is often complicated by prior attempts to repair the defect directly.

The MFC approach with binocular microscope provides excellent visualization of the lateral skull base and direct surgical access to the SCD, which is essential to ensuring adequate repair of the entire defect. However, a subset of patients with SCDS has unfavorable skull base topography and visualizing the defect under the microscopic is challenging (**Fig. 2**). Rigid endoscopes provide a superior view of the medial skull base and defects "hidden" from the microscopic view (**Fig. 3**). We now favor a small craniotomy approach for SCD repairs using endoscopes as an adjunct when necessary. This article discusses (1) the diagnosis of SCD, (2) the preoperative evaluation of SCD with an emphasis on patient selection and radiologic classification, (3) the MEEI endoscopic-assisted surgical technique to repair SCD via MFC, and (4) pearls and pitfalls with this approach.

DIAGNOSIS OF SUPERIOR CANAL DEHISCENCE

The diagnosis of SCDS encompasses a detailed clinical history, comprehensive head and neck examination, audiometric testing (with stapedius reflex), vestibular evoked myogenic potential (VEMP) testing, and high-resolution temporal bone computed tomography (CT).[9,25] Differential diagnoses to consider include otitis media with effusion, vestibular migraines, Meniere disease, benign paroxysmal positional vertigo, and patulous eustachian tube dysfunction.[26] If the patient has unilateral SCDS (or a less symptomatic contralateral ear), 512-Hz tuning fork testing usually lateralizes to the affected ear. The Dix-Hallpike test is typically normal unless the patient also has benign paroxysmal positional vertigo. Loud sounds (eg, from a Barany noise box), pneumatic otoscopy (or formal fistula testing), and Valsalva maneuver may trigger nystagmus, which can be enhanced by using Frenzel goggles to suppress visual fixation.

Audiometric Testing

Pure tone audiometry is an important component of the diagnostic work-up and should always include stapedial reflex testing, and bone conduction (BC) thresholds at −5 and −10 dB to test for "supranormal" bone conduction.[3] A low frequency (<2 kHz) air-bone gap of 20 to 30 dB caused by a combination of increased air conduction (AC) hearing threshold and supranormal BC threshold is typical.[27] Stapedius reflex testing is important because it can help separate SCDS from ossicular fixation or discontinuity, which can both cause low-frequency air-bone gap in the absence of overt middle ear disease on otoscopy examination.[11] In SCDS, the stapedius reflex is usually present, but absent in ossicular fixation (eg, otosclerosis) and ossicular discontinuity (unless the disruption is proximal to the stapedial tendon).[28]

Vestibular Evoked Myogenic Potential

Cervical (cVEMP) or ocular (oVEMP) VEMP are essential diagnostic tests in the assessment of patients suspected to have SCDS.[9,29] cVEMPs test the vestibulospinal reflex mediated through the saccule and the inferior vestibular nerve. A loud auditory stimulus induces an ipsilateral inhibition to the tonic sternocleidomastoid muscle activity recorded on an electromyogram. oVEMP (invoked by head tap or AC sound stimulus) is an excitatory electromyography response of the contralateral inferior oblique muscle and is driven by utricular otolith activation and superior vestibular nerve via the vestibulo-ocular pathway.[30] In SCDS, patients have abnormally low thresholds on cVEMP testing and elevated amplitudes on oVEMP testing. This is thought to reflect increased transmission of pressure through the vestibule. However, not all patients with symptomatic SCD have abnormal VEMP findings.[9]

Diagnostic Imaging

High-resolution CT imaging of the temporal bone is key in the diagnosis and surgical planning of SCD repair.[31] CT scans are known to overestimate the presence of SCD because very thin bone over the superior canal can appear absent.[32–35] To improve interpretation of CT scans for SCD, in addition to coronal and axial views, CT images should be reformatted to include Pöschl ("P" for parallel to superior canal, see **Fig. 1**) and Stenvers (transverse view of superior canal) views, which offer additions angles to examining the superior canal.[36] MRI of the brain may be obtained to rule out central causes of vestibular symptoms and to assess the intracranial anatomy along the skull base because middle fossa neoplasm have been found eroding into the superior canal in rare cases.[37]

ROLE OF ENDOSCOPE IN MIDDLE FOSSA CRANIOTOMY APPROACH SUPERIOR CANAL DEHISCENCE REPAIR

The goal of the MFC approach is to provide adequate exposure of the lateral skull base and visualization of the arcuate eminence while avoiding injury to brain, facial nerve, and any exposed ossicles from associated tegmental defects. Binocular microscopy provides a high-resolution, magnified view of the surgical field and confers the ability to perform two-handed surgery, but visualization of deeper recesses of the skull base

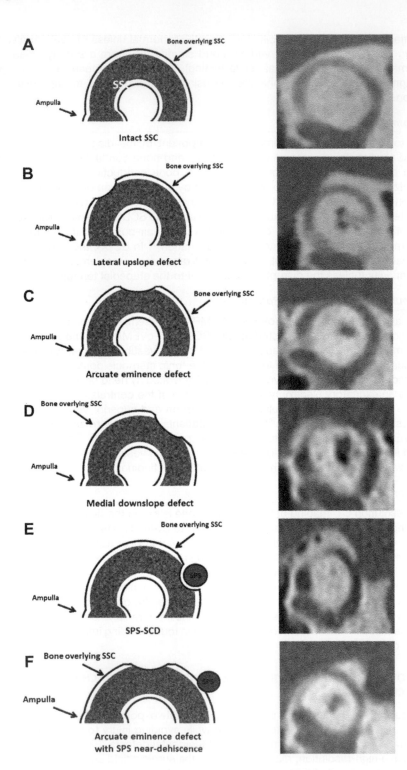

A — Intact SSC

B — Lateral upslope defect

C — Arcuate eminence defect

D — Medial downslope defect

E — SPS-SCD

F — Arcuate eminence defect with SPS near-dehiscence

Defect at peak of arcuate eminence
Easily visualized with microscope

Defect along medial downsloping tegmen
Not visible with microscope

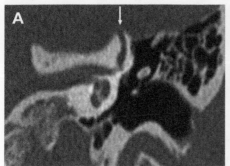
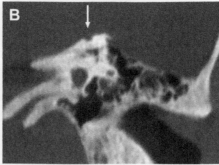

Fig. 2. Anatomic location of superior canal dehiscence on preoperative computed tomography scans can help anticipate the need for the endoscope during middle fossa craniotomy repair. High-resolution computed tomography: coronal views of temporal bone. (*A*) Defect is located at the peak of the arcuate eminence (*arrow*). Middle fossa craniotomy using the binocular microscope should provide adequate visualization of the entire defect. (*B*) Defect along the downsloping tegmen medial to the peak of the arcuate eminence (*arrow*). Microscopy could not visualize any portion of this defect. A 30° endoscope was used to identify and repair the dehiscence in this case. (*From* Carter MS, Lookabaugh S, Lee DJ. Endoscopic-assisted repair of superior canal dehiscence syndrome. Laryngoscope 2014;124(6):1465; with permission.)

is limited. The optical properties of a microscope necessitate an unobstructed view for adequate radiant exposure to illuminate the surgical plane. Moreover, areas of the middle fossa floor that are parallel to the microscope's visual axis do not reflect sufficient light back to the surgeon through the lenses and are therefore challenging to visualize.

A traditional microscope approach is acceptable for most SCD repairs, but some defects are hidden from the microscopic view (see **Fig. 2**). Specifically, defects along the medial downsloping tegmen and the posteromedial nonampullated end of the superior canal (see **Fig. 1**C) can be obscured from microscopic view. Before incorporating the endoscope, these defects were addressed with a large craniotomy, extensive temporal lobe retraction, and were repaired after drilling the lateral skull base ridge and/or applying bone wax blindly along that predicted location of the SCD. Partial visualization of the defect increases the risk of an inadequate repair,

---

Fig. 1. Radiologic classification of patients with SCD based on defect location. (*Left column*) Schematic of defect location relative to the ampullated end of the superior canal. (*Right Column*) Computed tomography images in the plane of Pöschl of corresponding defects. (*A*) Intact superior semicircular canal (SSC). (*B*) Dehiscence near the ampullated end of the SSC, often on the lateral upslope of the arcuate eminence. (*C*) Dehiscence of the superior tip of the SSC, corresponding with the peak of the arcuate eminence. (*D*) Dehiscence along the posterior limb of the superior canal, often on the medial downslope of the arcuate eminence. (*E*) Superior petrosal sinus (SPS)-associated SCD. (*F*) An unusual case of two dehiscences along a single superior canal: arcuate eminence defect with a "near dehiscence" SSC associated with the SPS. (*Adapted from* Lookabaugh S, Kelly HR, Carter MS, et al. Radiologic classification of superior canal dehiscence: implications for surgical repair. Otol Neurotol 2015;36(1):120; with permission.)

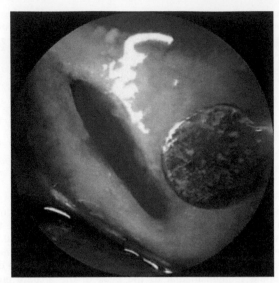

Fig. 3. Intraoperative image of arcuate eminence defect with a 30° endoscope following middle fossa craniotomy. Right ear, 30° endoscopy demonstrates an arcuate eminence bony defect. Note the blue-lined region toward the ampulla (*upper left*) and exposure of the endosteum and/or the membranous labyrinth of the arcuate eminence. The Rosen knife in the image is 2 mm in diameter. (*Adapted from* Carter MS, Lookabaugh S, Lee DJ. Endoscopic-assisted repair of superior canal dehiscence syndrome. Laryngoscope 2014;124(6):1467; with permission.)

and experimental studies have suggested that small gaps in SCD repairs may result in the failure to restore normal physiology,[4,38] which would likely be perceived clinically as persistent symptoms. The endoscope enables smaller diameter craniotomies, whereas improved visualization limits retraction of the brain and drilling near the inner ear by taking advantage of the angled endoscopes to look beyond the arcuate eminence (see **Fig. 3**; **Fig. 4**).

Additionally, in some cases, patients diagnosed with SCDS may have an apparent bony defect on preoperative CT, but a "near dehiscence" or "blue lined" superior canal is revealed intraoperatively during MFC SCD repair (**Fig. 5**). These areas of thin bone over the superior canal can be difficult to locate using the binocular microscope given the surrounding tegmen defects and lack of landmarks that often accompany most lateral skull base explorations. With the lens and light source at the distal tip, endoscopes are particularly helpful in locating blue-lined SCDs because they provide a greater high-definition (HD) view and better transillumination of the skull base.

PREOPERATIVE PLANNING

Recently, we proposed a formal MEEI radiologic classification system for SCD that was designed with surgical planning in mind (**Box 1**).[39] The system relies on high-resolution CT imaging and highlights surgically relevant skull base morphology, including the position of the SCD along the middle fossa floor (see **Figs. 1** and **2**), and the radiologic appearance of the tegmen and facial nerve.[40] The key feature to consider in the discussion of endoscopic-guided SCD repairs is the anatomic location of the SCD relative to the peak of the arcuate eminence and the slope of the tegmen floor (see **Fig. 2**).[40] Most SCDs are on the arcuate eminence (59.2%) or lateral to the

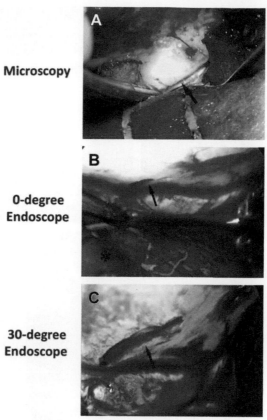

Fig. 4. Intraoperative images during middle fossa craniotomy and SCD surgery, left ear. (*A*) Binocular microscopy in the region of the arcuate eminence (*arrow*) and petrous ridge following middle fossa craniotomy. The SCD was not seen. A middle fossa retractor is used to maintain surgical exposure. (*B*) In the left ear, improved view of the ampullated half of the superior canal defect using 0° endoscopy (*arrow*). The temporal lobe (*asterisk*) is gently retracted to expose the SCD. (*C*) In the left ear, both the ampullated and nonampullated ends of the dehiscence are seen with a 3-mm, 30° rigid endoscope, defining the exact limits of this arcuate eminence defect (*arrow*). (*Adapted from* Carter MS, Lookabaugh S, Lee DJ. Endoscopic-assisted repair of superior canal dehiscence syndrome. Laryngoscope 2014;124(6):1467; with permission.)

peak of the arcuate eminence on the upsloping tegmen (7.6%), and are therefore amenable to direct visualization and access via MFC approach using the microscope with minimal retraction of the temporal lobe.[39] In contrast, SCDs that are medial to the peak of arcuate eminence (see **Fig. 2**B) fall along the downsloping tegmen (29.8%) and are often obscured from direct view through the binocular microscope (see **Fig. 4**).

Facial nerve complications can arise following MFC and skull base dissection because patients with SCD are more likely to have a dehiscent geniculate ganglion.[41] Previous radiographic studies, including studies from our group, have found that nearly 50% of patients with SCD have exposed geniculate ganglions.[39,41] Isaacson and Vrabec[41] highlighted that a dehiscent geniculate ganglion may be obscured from view during MFC because of irregular tegmen topography, consequently increasing the risk of iatrogenic injury. Preoperative knowledge of a dehiscent

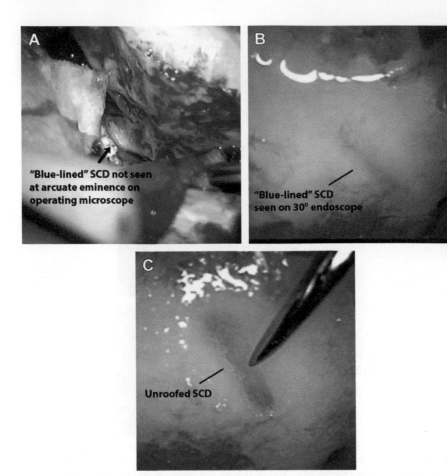

Fig. 5. Intraoperative images of blue-lined SCD surgery, right ear. (*A*) Binocular microscopy in the region of the arcuate eminence (*arrow*) following middle fossa craniotomy. The canal defect was not seen. (*B*) In the right ear, improved view of the middle fossa floor using 30° endoscopy reveals area of thin bone over superior canal. (*C*) In the right ear, thin bone over the arcuate eminence has been removed using a 1.5-mm diamond burr at low speed (5000 rpm). This defect was then occluded with bone wax (not shown).

geniculate ganglion is therefore essential and careful anterior dissection along the skull base following the petrous ridge with continuous facial nerve monitoring and endoscopic-guidance can reduce the risk of injury.[39]

MASSACHUSETTS EYE AND EAR INFIRMARY ENDOSCOPIC-ASSISTED REPAIR OF SUPERIOR CANAL DEHISCENCE

We began using the endoscope for MFC SCD repairs in 2013 and have used the endoscope in most cases (29 out of 45) performed at MEEI since.[40] Our experience with endoscopic-assisted SCD repair is summarized in **Table 1**. All patients were adults (18 years or older) with CT-confirmed SCD and intolerable auditory and/or vestibular symptoms, and audiometric and cVEMP testing consistent with symptomatic SCD. CT scans are evaluated based on the MEEI SCD radiologic classification system,[39]

Box 1
Radiologic classification of superior canal dehiscence: CT characteristics

1. Dehiscence of the superior semicircular canal (SSC)
   a. Intact SSC: bone overlying SSC in all slices in all views/reformats
   b. Near dehiscence: thin bone overlying the SSC or dehiscence apparent in only *one* slice in one view/reformat
   c. Frank dehiscence: obvious lack of bone overlying SSC in *at least two* consecutive slices in at least one view/reformat

2. Tegmen dehiscence
   a. Lack of bone *without* soft tissue opacification in middle ear cavity
   b. Lack of bone *with* soft tissue opacification in middle ear cavity; *no* ossicular contact
   c. Lack of bone *with* soft tissue opacification in middle ear cavity; *with* ossicular contact
   d. Intact tegmen

3. Low-lying tegmen
   In the coronal view, angle measured from vertical line through SSC:
   a. 75° or greater: flat/not low-lying
   b. 74° or less: low-lying

4. Geniculate ganglion dehiscence
   In the coronal view, definite lack of bone over geniculate ganglion on at least two consecutive slices

5. Superior petrosal sinus associated SCD
   Where superior petrosal sinus can clearly be distinguished by a bony groove in the petrous bone and juxtaposed to the site of SCD

6. Estimated location of the SCD
   Linear distance measured in the coronal view from the outer table of temporal bone to center of the SCD

Adapted from Lookabaugh S, Kelly HR, Carter MS, et al. Radiologic classification of superior canal dehiscence: implications for surgical repair. Otol Neurotol 2015;36(1):124; with permission.

Table 1
Overview of experience: MFC endoscopic-assisted SCD repairs

MFC approach SCD repairs	
Total number (microscope only and endoscope-assisted) since 2013	45 cases
Endoscope-assisted repairs	29 cases
Gender	13 males, 14 females (2 had bilateral repairs)
Side of repair	13 left, 16 right
Revision SCD surgery	4/29
Able to visualize entire SCD	29/29
Facial palsy or cerebrospinal fluid leak	0/29

We first started using endoscopes in MFC SCD repairs in February 2013. Out of 45 MFC SCD repairs performed since then, 29 cases were endoscope-assisted. The microscope was deemed adequate for the remaining cases. The 29 endoscope-assisted cases were performed on 27 patients. Two patients had bilateral sequential repairs (12 months apart).

and patients with defects along a medial downsloping tegmen (see **Fig. 2**B) are flagged for endoscopic-assisted repairs if the MFC approach is deemed to be most appropriate.

Endoscopes allow rapid localization of blue-lined superior canals because the distal endoscopic light source transilluminates the middle fossa floor (see **Fig. 5**). Symptomatic "near dehiscence" superior canals may then be unroofed gently and occluded with autologous tissue or bone wax. The decision to unroof "near dehiscence" superior canals is based on the finding that resurfacing areas of thin bone is associated with poor symptom resolution or rapid recurrence of symptoms.[42]

An endoscopic view also improves identification of a dehiscent geniculate ganglion, helping to prevent inadvertent injury to the facial nerve. We have had no facial nerve palsies or postoperative cerebral spinal fluid leaks in all 29 cases of endoscopic-guided MFC SCD repairs and in all cases, a superior visualization of the entire defect (compared with the binocular microscope) was achieved.

ENDOSCOPIC EQUIPMENT

Standard equipment needed for endoscopic ear surgery includes a light source and rigid endoscope coupled to a three-CCD, HD camera and HD video monitor. Currently, the Hopkins rod-lens system is a popular choice among otolaryngologists and provides endoscopes of varying diameters, lengths, and angles of view. The rigid endoscope diameters commonly used for ear surgery are 2.7, 3.0, and 4.0 mm. Endoscopes with larger diameter transmit more light to the operative field, and thus the image quality improves. Wider diameter endoscopes, however, decrease the working space available to maneuver surgical instruments. Typical endoscope shaft lengths in middle ear surgery are 11, 14, and 18 cm. The angles of view most commonly used are 0° and 30° angled endoscopes. We routinely use a 3.0-mm diameter, 14-cm Hopkins rod for our transcanal ear cases and lateral skull base surgery.

In addition to rigid endoscope choices, light of varying brightness and quality is offered by three different types of light sources: halogen, xenon, and LED. Xenon light sources are standard for sinus surgery and available at most institutions. The light source should be set at no more than 50% intensity to reduce heat exposure to surrounding tissues.[43]

There is a host of commercially available surgical endoscopic equipment. Because endoscopic ear surgery is still in its infancy, these instruments are undergoing continual evaluation and refinement. At the very minimum, defogging solution and microwipe are needed for cleaning the lens of the endoscope and a suction-dissector to enable one-handed dissection. Finally, the room setup should include a binocular microscope and standard otologic instrument sets.

SURGICAL OVERVIEW OF ENDOSCOPIC-ASSISTED MIDDLE FOSSA CRANIOTOMY SUPERIOR CANAL DEHISCENCE REPAIR

The patient is positioned supine, with the anesthesiologist on the same side as the surgeon and the scrub team placed opposite the surgeon before the start of the case. Positioning the operating microscope (with the binocular teaching head mounted on the side ipsilateral to the surgical ear) and endoscope setup before the patient is brought into the room allows for the HD monitor to be placed ideally in front of the surgeon at eye-level and at the foot of the bed, opposite the ear to be operated on (**Fig. 6**). Following intubation and a minimal hair shave, a 6 to 7 cm curvilinear incision is drawn, extending from 1 cm posterior and superior to the postauricular skin crease and curving anteriorly along the floor of the middle fossa and superiorly over the temporalis

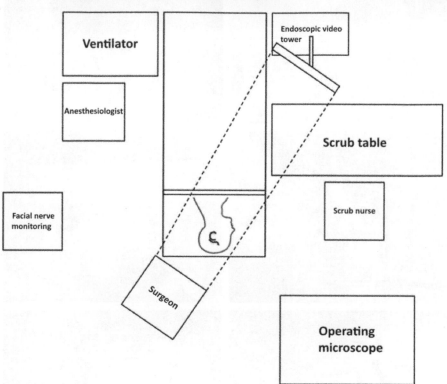

Fig. 6. Operating room (OR) setup for endoscopic-assisted middle fossa craniotomy and superior canal dehiscence repair on the left ear. The high-definition video tower (or boom-mounted video screen) is placed directly opposite the surgeon for direct line of sight using rigid endoscopy at the foot of the bed. The scrub nurse is across from the surgeon. The microscope is placed to the right of the patient's head and is brought in as needed. Anesthesia is at the foot of the bed on the same side as the surgeon. (*Adapted from* Carter MS, Lookabaugh S, Lee DJ. Endoscopic-assisted repair of superior canal dehiscence syndrome. Laryngoscope 2014;124(6):1466; with permission.)

towards the hairline anteriorly (**Fig. 7**A). This approach avoids the need for a preauricular incision and associated cosmetic deformity of a linear incision. A total of 10 to 15 mL of 1% lidocaine with 1:100,000 epinephrine is infiltrated into the planned surgical field. The ear is then prepared and draped in the usual sterile fashion. Continuous facial nerve monitoring is used routinely for all lateral skull base surgery at MEEI.

The skin incision is then made parallel to the hair follicle roots to reduce the risk of alopecia along the surgical scar. The incision is made approximately 1 cm above the attachment of the pinna superiorly to avoid discomfort with wearing glasses that fall on the scar line postoperatively. Care is taken to not extend the incision past the anterior hairline. The skin flaps are elevated superficially to the temporalis fascia sharply (**Fig. 7**B). Bipolar cautery is favored for focal hemostasis. Sharp and blunt dissection is used whenever possible with avoidance of monopolar cautery when possible. A

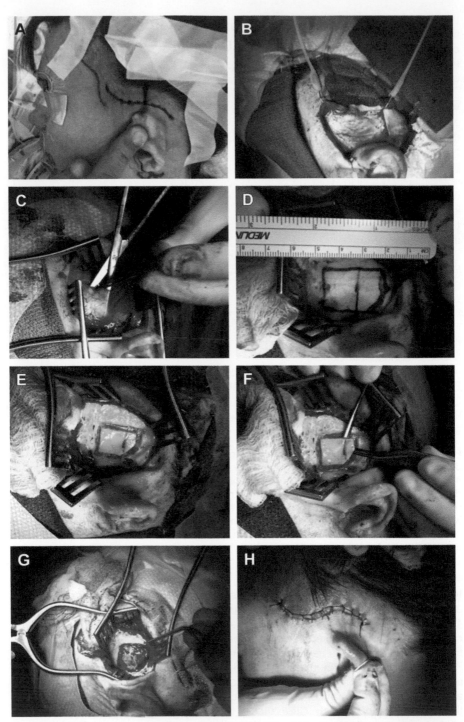

Fig. 7. Montage of surgical approach. (*A*) A 6- to 7-cm curvilinear Incision is drawn, extending from 1 cm posterior and superior to the postauricular skin crease and curving anteriorly along the floor of the middle fossa and superiorly over the temporalis into the hairline

temporalis fascia graft is harvested centrally (**Fig. 7**C), allowing for a peripheral rim of fascia to facilitate closure. An anteroinferiorly based muscle and periosteal flap is designed, carried down to the bone, and elevated anteriorly and inferiorly to expose the bony external auditory meatus. An inferiorly based temporalis muscle flap is associated with greater pain issue postoperatively.

A 2 × 3 cm bone flap is marked and centered on the external auditory canal (**Fig. 7**D) with the inferior extent just above the bony meatus and the mastoid prominence to avoid exposing air cells. The bone flap is elevated using cutting and diamond drill burrs (**Fig. 7**E, F). The dura is gently elevated off the tegmen mastoideum and tegmen tympani. Careful attention is paid to dissecting the middle fossa dura from posterior to anterior until the region of the arcuate eminence is visualized. Use of a fenestrated suction tip is crucial to avoid suctioning over an exposed superior canal. The tegmen is often thin or dehiscent and can make the initial survey to localize the SCD challenging in some cases. The distance from the outer table of cranium to the SCD (highlighted in the MEEI SCD radiologic classification scheme[39]) on a coronal-view CT is a useful measurement to make preoperatively that is used to approximate the location of the SCD during surgery. Once the SCD is identified, a middle fossa retractor is placed. When the defect is not visualized by standard microscopy either because of its anatomic location (medial downsloping tegmen) or if there is difficulty visualizing a blue-lined or near dehiscence, the endoscope is brought into the operating field. At this point, a 3.0-mm diameter, 14-cm-long 0°, 30°, or 45° endoscope is introduced into the craniotomy and stabilized with the nondominant hand to provide a view of the skull base (see **Fig. 4**).

Under endoscopic control, the dura is dissected from the medial aspect of the defect. For a blue-lined superior canal, a 1.5-mm diamond burr at low speed (5000 RPM) is used under endoscopic visualization to unroof the defect to the endosteum layer (see **Fig. 5**). After exposing the defect, occlusion of the defect is gently performed using surgical bone wax. The wax is applied using either a round knife or Freer elevator. An assistant may hold a fenestrated suction near the region of (but not directly on) the defect to help clear the irrigation fluid and blood. The repair is then irrigated under direct visualization to ensure stability of the bone wax. Using human temporal bones, we have demonstrated that very small volumes of wax result in complete occlusion the canal.[44] Addition applications of wax encourage extension of wax along the superior canal lumen toward the ampulla and the common crus and could result in vestibular dysfunction or hearing loss.

If the exposed tegmen is dehiscent, a split calvarial bone chip wrapped in temporalis fascia is used to repair the skull base. Wounds are closed in a layered watertight fashion with no drain and a mastoid dressing is applied for 5 days (**Fig. 7**G, H). At our institution, all patients are admitted postoperatively to a monitored care setting overnight. The average hospital stay is approximately 2 days.

SUMMARY

Intraoperative use of the rigid endoscope during MFC is a safe and provides an effective adjunct to the microscope to identify and repair cases of SCD that are hidden from

---

anteriorly. (*B*) An anteriorly based muscle and periosteal flap is designed. (*C*) Temporalis fascia harvest. (*D–G*) A 2 cm × 3 cm bone flap is marked and centered on the external auditory canal. The bone flap is elevated using cutting and diamond drill burrs. (*H*) Wounds are closed in a layered fashion with no drain and a mastoid dressing is applied for 5 days.

line of sight surgery. The endoscope improves visualization of the entire dehiscence and provides better transillumination of the skull base when localizing a blue-lined defect. The approach also reduces the extent and duration of temporal lobe retraction.

Disadvantages of using endoscopy during MFC include the need for one-handed dissection and a poor depth perception in comparison with the microscope. Consequently, the surgeon must be experienced with the endoscope to appropriately determine the depth of the operative site. However, the benefits of an endoscope-assisted SCD repair in appropriate cases where the defect cannot be clearly visualized because of skull base variability outweigh these disadvantages. Refinements in endoscope holders, combination suction-dissector instrumentation, the use of an endoscopic lens scrubber, and the introduction of three-dimensional endoscopy will address some of these limitations.

REFERENCES

1. Minor LB, Solomon D, Zinreich JS, et al. Sound- and/or pressure-induced vertigo due to bone dehiscence of the superior semicircular canal. Arch Otolaryngol Head Neck Surg 1998;124(3):249–58.

2. Minor LB. Clinical manifestations of superior semicircular canal dehiscence. Laryngoscope 2005;115(10):1717–27.

3. Merchant SN, Rosowski JJ. Conductive hearing loss caused by third-window lesions of the inner ear. Otol Neurotol 2008;29(3):282–9.

4. Pisano DV, Niesten ME, Merchant SN, et al. The effect of superior semicircular canal dehiscence on intracochlear sound pressures. Audiol Neurootol 2012;17(5): 338–48.

5. Rosowski JJ, Songer JE, Nakajima HH, et al. Clinical, experimental, and theoretical investigations of the effect of superior semicircular canal dehiscence on hearing mechanisms. Otol Neurotol 2004;25(3):323–32.

6. Migliaccio AA, Minor LB, Carey JP. Vergence-mediated modulation of the human angular vestibulo-ocular reflex is unaffected by canal plugging. Exp Brain Res 2008;186(4):581–7.

7. Kim N, Steele CR, Puria S. Superior-semicircular-canal dehiscence: effects of location, shape, and size on sound conduction. Hear Res 2013;301:72–84.

8. Songer JE, Rosowski JJ. A superior semicircular canal dehiscence-induced air-bone gap in chinchilla. Hear Res 2010;269(1–2):70–80.

9. Niesten ME, McKenna MJ, Herrmann BS, et al. Utility of cVEMPs in bilateral superior canal dehiscence syndrome. Laryngoscope 2013;123(1):226–32.

10. Welgampola MS, Migliaccio AA, Myrie OA, et al. The human sound-evoked vestibulo-ocular reflex and its electromyographic correlate. Clin Neurophysiol 2009; 120(1):158–66.

11. Cox KM, Lee DJ, Carey JP, et al. Dehiscence of bone overlying the superior semicircular canal as a cause of an air-bone gap on audiometry: a case study. Am J Audiol 2003;12(1):11–6.

12. Jung DH, Lookabaugh SA, Owoc MS, et al. Dizziness is more prevalent than autophony among patients who have undergone repair of superior canal dehiscence. Otol Neurotol 2015;36:126–32.

13. Remenschneider AK, Owoc M, Kozin ED, et al. Health utility improves after surgery for superior canal dehiscence syndrome. Otol Neurotol 2015;36(10): 1695–701.

14. Gioacchini FM, Alicandri-Ciufelli M, Kaleci S, et al. Outcomes and complications in superior semicircular canal dehiscence surgery: a systematic review. Laryngoscope 2016;126(5):1218–24.
15. Vlastarakos PV, Proikas K, Tavoulari E, et al. Efficacy assessment and complications of surgical management for superior semicircular canal dehiscence: a meta-analysis of published interventional studies. Eur Arch Otorhinolaryngol 2009;266(2):177–86.
16. Amoodi HA, Makki FM, McNeil M, et al. Transmastoid resurfacing of superior semicircular canal dehiscence. Laryngoscope 2011;121(5):1117–23.
17. Crovetto M, Areitio E, Elexpuru J, et al. Transmastoid approach for resurfacing of superior semicircular canal dehiscence. Auris Nasus Larynx 2008;35(2):247–9.
18. Fiorino F, Barbieri F, Pizzini FB, et al. A dehiscent superior semicircular canal may be plugged and resurfaced via the transmastoid route. Otol Neurotol 2010;31(1): 136–9.
19. Lundy L, Zapala D, Moushey J. Cartilage cap occlusion technique for dehiscent superior semicircular canals. Otol Neurotol 2011;32(8):1281–4.
20. Teixido M, Seymour PE, Kung B, et al. Transmastoid middle fossa craniotomy repair of superior semicircular canal dehiscence using a soft tissue graft. Otol Neurotol 2011;32(5):877–81.
21. Van Haesendonck G, Van de Heyning P, Van Rompaey V. Retrospective cohort study on hearing outcome after transmastoid plugging in superior semicircular canal dehiscence syndrome. Clin Otolaryngol 2015. [Epub ahead of print].
22. Agrawal SK, Parnes LS. Transmastoid superior semicircular canal occlusion. Otol Neurotol 2008;29(3):363–7.
23. Teixido MT, Artz GJ, Kung BC. Clinical experience with symptomatic superior canal dehiscence in a single neurotologic practice. Otolaryngol Head Neck Surg 2008;139(3):405–13.
24. McCall AA, McKenna MJ, Merchant SN, et al. Superior canal dehiscence syndrome associated with the superior petrosal sinus in pediatric and adult patients. Otol Neurotol 2011;32(8):1312–9.
25. Niesten ME, Hamberg LM, Silverman JB, et al. Superior canal dehiscence length and location influences clinical presentation and audiometric and cervical vestibular-evoked myogenic potential testing. Audiol Neurootol 2014;19(2): 97–105.
26. Lempert T, von Brevern M. Episodic vertigo. Curr Opin Neurol 2005;18(1):5–9.
27. McEvoy TP, Mikulec AA, Armbrecht ES, et al. Quantification of hearing loss associated with superior semi-circular canal dehiscence. Am J Otolaryngol 2013; 34(4):345–9.
28. Mikulec AA, McKenna MJ, Ramsey MJ, et al. Superior semicircular canal dehiscence presenting as conductive hearing loss without vertigo. Otol Neurotol 2004; 25(2):121–9.
29. Zuniga M, Janky K. Ocular vs. cervical VEMPs in the diagnosis of superior semicircular canal dehiscence syndrome. Otol Neurotol 2013;34(1):121–6.
30. Janky KL, Nguyen KD, Welgampola M, et al. Air-conducted oVEMPs provide the best separation between intact and superior canal dehiscent labyrinths. Otol Neurotol 2013;34(1):127–34.
31. Curtin HD. Imaging of conductive hearing loss with a normal tympanic membrane. AJR Am J Roentgenol 2016;206(1):49–56.
32. Eibenberger K, Carey J, Ehtiati T, et al. A novel method of 3D image analysis of high-resolution cone beam CT and multi slice CT for the detection of semicircular canal dehiscence. Otol Neurotol 2014;35(2):329–37.

33. Stimmer H, Hamann KF, Zeiter S, et al. Semicircular canal dehiscence in HR multi-slice computed tomography: distribution, frequency, and clinical relevance. Eur Arch Otorhinolaryngol 2012;269(2):475–80.

34. Elmali M, Polat AV, Kucuk H, et al. Semicircular canal dehiscence: frequency and distribution on temporal bone CT and its relationship with the clinical outcomes. Eur J Radiol 2013;82(10):e606–9.

35. Cloutier JF, Belair M, Saliba I. Superior semicircular canal dehiscence: positive predictive value of high-resolution CT scanning. Eur Arch Otorhinolaryngol 2008;265(12):1455–60.

36. Belden CJ, Weg N, Minor LB, et al. CT evaluation of bone dehiscence of the superior semicircular canal as a cause of sound- and/or pressure-induced vertigo. Radiology 2003;226(2):337–43.

37. Crane BT, Carey JP, McMenomey S, et al. Meningioma causing superior canal dehiscence syndrome. Otol Neurotol 2010;31(6):1009–10.

38. Brockenbrough JM, Marzo S, Wurster R, et al. Bone wax prevents nystagmus after labyrinthine fenestration in guinea pigs. Otolaryngol Head Neck Surg 2003; 128(5):726–31.

39. Lookabaugh S, Kelly HR, Carter MS, et al. Radiologic classification of superior canal dehiscence: implications for surgical repair. Otol Neurotol 2015;36(1): 118–25.

40. Carter MS, Lookabaugh S, Lee DJ. Endoscopic-assisted repair of superior canal dehiscence syndrome. Laryngoscope 2014;124(6):1464–8.

41. Isaacson B, Vrabec JT. The radiographic prevalence of geniculate ganglion dehiscence in normal and congenitally thin temporal bones. Otol Neurotol 2007;28(1):107–10.

42. Ward BK, Wenzel A, Ritzl EK, et al. Near-dehiscence: clinical findings in patients with thin bone over the superior semicircular canal. Otol Neurotol 2013;34(8): 1421–8.

43. Kozin ED, Lehmann A, Carter M, et al. Thermal effects of endoscopy in a human temporal bone model: implications for endoscopic ear surgery. Laryngoscope 2014;124(8):1–8.

44. Cheng YS, Kozin ED, Remenschneider AK, et al. Characteristics of wax occlusion in the surgical repair of superior canal dehiscence in human temporal bone specimens. Otol Neurotol 2016;37(1):83–8.

Endoscopic Management of Middle Ear and Temporal Bone Lesions

Brandon Isaacson, MD, FACS[a],*, João Flávio Nogueira, MD[b]

KEYWORDS

- Endoscopic ear surgery • Paraganglioma • Glomus tympanicum
- Middle ear adenoma • Cholesterol granuloma • Petrous apex • Temporal bone
- Skull base

KEY POINTS

- Middle ear paraganglioma is a benign neoplasm that typically presents with vascular tinnitus and progressive hearing loss depending on the size and location of the tumor.
- Petrous apex cholesterol granuloma is a cystic, inflammatory lesion typically resulting from hemorrhage into a mucosalized space; they can managed with marsupialization into the middle ear or mastoid in symptomatic patients.
- Middle ear adenoma is a benign but locally aggressive lesion that has a high incidence of recurrence without complete surgical excision.
- Transcanal endoscopic ear surgery is a means of managing temporal bone neoplasms given the unparalleled visualization of the tumor's relationship to the critical anatomic structures within the lateral skull base.

INTRODUCTION

Lesions involving the temporal bone, although rare, are often a challenge to manage given the adjacent critical structures that are localized within the skull base. Fortunately, most lesions involving the middle ear and mastoid are benign, thus obviating the need to obtain the wide tissue margins that would typically result in significant morbidity. The microscopic transcanal or postauricular approaches are the traditional means to excise lesions of the middle ear and mastoid. Transcanal endoscopic ear surgery (TEES) is a relatively new option that can be used to address pathology of

Disclosures: Advanced Bionics – Medical Advisory Board and Consultant, Stryker – Course Instructor, Medtronic – Consultant.
[a] Department of Otolaryngology – Head and Neck Surgery, University of Texas Southwestern Medical Center, 5323 Harry Hines Boulevard, Dallas, TX 75390-9035, USA; [b] Hospital Geral de Fortaleza, Fortaleza, Brazil
* Corresponding author.
E-mail address: Brandon.isaacson@utsouthwestern.edu

Otolaryngol Clin N Am 49 (2016) 1205–1214
http://dx.doi.org/10.1016/j.otc.2016.05.011
oto.theclinics.com
0030-6665/16/$ – see front matter © 2016 Elsevier Inc. All rights reserved.

the middle ear and mastoid.[1] TEES uses the ear canal as the access point to address pathology of the temporal bone. The endoscope, unlike the microscope, is not limited by line of site issues and allows for improved illumination of the surgical field. The endoscope provides a wide field view that allows the surgeon to examine areas not typically visible with the microscope without removal of bone lateral to the area of interest.[2] The endoscope also does not require a postauricular incision, which results in less postoperative pain and allows for a faster recovery. Disadvantages of TEES include moving from 2-handed to 1-handed tissue dissection, and the lack of depth perception. This article describes the usefulness of TEES for the management of temporal bone lesions including middle ear paragangliomas (MEPs), adenoma, petrous apex cholesterol granuloma (PACG), and other lesions.

TECHNIQUE

The patient is positioned 90° to 180° away from anesthesia after induction and intubation. Total intravenous anesthesia is the technique of choice because it reduces the chance of patent movement, does not require muscle relaxants, and is reported to reduce intraoperative bleeding. A 3-mm diameter 14-cm length endoscope with varying degrees of angulation (0°, 30°, 45°, 70°) and a high-definition 3-chip camera are the ideal equipment for TEES. Local anesthesia with lidocaine or bupivacaine with epinephrine is infiltrated into the membranous canal skin, tragus, and postauricular area, which can be done with the microscope and a speculum or with the endoscope without a speculum. Excess hair in the membranous canal is trimmed to prevent smearing of blood and irrigation on the tip of the endoscope. Topical 1:1000 epinephrine on cotton or 0.025- by 0.25-inch cottonoids can be placed on the medial canal skin and tympanic membrane, which helps to reduce bleeding. The extent and location of middle ear pathology dictates the type of canal incisions that are made.

A standard tympanomeatal flap is elevated for pathology located posterior to the annulus, which typically entails incisions that are just anterior to the level of the lateral process of the malleus superiorly and at the 6 o'clock position inferiorly. The inferior and posterior osseous annulus can be removed with a drill or curette to provide additional exposure of the hypotympanum and retrotympanum. Angled endoscopes permit visualization of anterior, superior, posterior, or inferior extensions of disease that often obviates the need for additional bone removal. Bone removal may be required in some cases to allow for instrument and suction access to the pathology.[3]

Three TEES approach options are available for lesions localized anterior to the malleus, or within the petrous apex. Malleus degloving necessitates a wider tympanomeatal flap with elevation of the tympanic membrane off the malleus lateral process, handle, and umbo. Malleus degloving provides excellent exposure to the anterior and posterior mesotympanum, but limited exposure of the protympanum if there is a prominent anterior canal wall bulge. This approach can also be used for the infracochlear approach to the petrous apex. Disadvantages of this approach are that a myringoplasty may be required, because a tear in the tympanic membrane may be difficult to avoid when elevating the drum off the umbo.[3]

A superiorly based tympanomeatal flap provides access to the entire hypotympanum, retrotympanum, and anterior mesotympanum. The canal incisions for the superiorly based tympanomeatal flap approach start at the level of the lateral process of the malleus and extends around the posterior canal wall along the inferior canal and up the anterior canal wall. The canal incision is typically made at least 7 mm lateral to the anterior, posterior, and inferior annulus to account for any additional removal of the inferior and posterior medial canal. The canal skin is then elevated down to the tympanic annulus and the fibrous annulus is elevated out of the annular sulcus. The tympanic membrane is left pedicled to the superior canal skin and the malleus. This approach provides wide access for the infracochlear approach to the petrous apex, and allows for excision of most middle ear tumors, which do not extend superior into the epitympanum. At the completion of tumor removal, the tympanomeatal flap is easily restored to its normal anatomic position, often without the need for a tissue graft.[3]

Ear canal and tympanic membrane degloving can be used for almost any lesion within the middle ear or medial temporal bone. In this approach, the osseous ear canal skin along with the entire tympanic membrane is removed after separating the drum from the malleus and the osseous annulus. A canaloplasty can then be performed to further enhance exposure to the entire middle ear and to more deep-seated lesions. Removal of the lateral chain with primary or delayed reconstruction can further enhance exposure. The canal skin and tympanic membrane can be replaced at the end of the procedure in addition to the use of a tissue graft if necessary. Patients with nonserviceable hearing can undergo blind sac closure with middle ear and Eustachian tube obliteration, which may be preferred in cases where entry into the subarachnoid space is required.[3]

MIDDLE EAR PARAGANGLIOMA

MEP, also known as glomus tympanicum, is a benign, slow-growing, vascular neoplasm that typically originates from the tympanic plexus of Arnold's and Jacobson's nerve along the cochlear promontory.[4] MEP is also the most common neoplasm that originate within the middle ear.[5] Histologically these tumors are composed of balls of chief cells (Zellballen formation) intermixed with sustentactular cells. MEPs have an identical appearance to their counterparts in other head and neck locations, including those lesions that arise from the carotid artery, jugular bulb, and vagus nerve.[6] Malignant and catecholamine-producing head and neck paragangliomas are rare and this is no exception for those that arise in the temporal bone.[7,8]

Paragangliomas are rare, and represent 1% of all tumors of the head and neck with the carotid body being the most common location.[9] A recent series of 115 patients confirmed that the vast majority of MEPs occur in females (90%). The mean age at time of diagnosis for MEPs was 55.2 years with a bimodal distribution in the late 30 s and the early 60 s.[10]

MEPs most commonly present with symptoms of hearing loss, pulsatile tinnitus, and ear fullness, although approximately 12% are incidentally identified on physical examination. These tumors rarely present with bloody otorrhea or cranial neuropathies.[10]

Surgical excision is the preferred management strategy for MEPs, although observation or radiation are also options in selected cases. Several staging systems (Fisch–Mattox, Sanna, Glasscock–Jackson; **Tables 1–3**), exist for describing the extent of MEPs, which uses both physical examination and imaging with either computed tomography or MRI (**Fig. 1**).[11–13]

A transcanal microscopic approach is typically favored for smaller tumors (Glasscock–Jackson stages I and II), whereas tumors that extend into the mastoid or into

Table 1 The Fisch–Mattox classification system	
Grade	Definition
A	Tumor entirely within the middle ear space
B	Tumor only within the middle ear or mastoid portion of the temporal bone
C	Tumor within the infralabyrinthine temporal bone or petrous apex
D1	Tumors with <2 cm of intracranial extension
D2	Tumors with ≥2 cm of intracranial extension

From Fisch U. Infratemporal fossa approach for extensive tumors of the temporal bone and base of skull. In: Silverstein H, Norrell H, editors. Neurological surgery of the ear. Birmingham (AL): Aesculapius; 1977. p. 34–53.

the ear canal (Glasscock–Jackson stages III or IV) are often managed with a postauricular transcanal transmastoid approach. Glasscock–Jackson stages I and II MEP in a patient with a small or narrow ear canal may necessitate to conversion to an open approach. MEPs with significant anterior extension into the protympanum, posterior extension into the retrotympanum (sinus tympani, sinus subtympanicum, facial recess), or inferior extension into the hypotympanum may also require a postauricular approach with the addition of a mastoidectomy to completely eradicate disease.[10]

TEES is suited uniquely to MEPs that extend to these locations because the wide field of view and angled endoscopes readily allow the surgeon to visualize and excise extensions of disease outside of the mesotympanum (**Fig. 2**). Marchioni and colleagues[14] reported using an exclusive TEES approach to completely excise 2 Fisch–Mattox stage B1 tumors, and 1 stage A1 tumor. The authors have removed 13 tumors, all of which were Fisch–Mattox stages A1 to B1, using the TEES approach. Ten of the 13 tumors were removed exclusively using the endoscope. The microscope was used in 3 cases. In 1 case, the microscope was used without a postauricular incision to control bleeding and to remove a small remnant of tumor in the hypotympanum. Two other patients required a postauricular incision with mastoidectomy to completely excise the tumor. No complications were noted in any of these procedures. No recurrences have been observed in the author's series of 13 patients; however, the follow-up duration for most patients is less than 1 year.

The advantages of TEES for the management of MEP include no need for a retroauricular incision, the ability to visualize and remove disease extensions into the protympanum, retrotympanum, and hypotympanum without excessive bone removal. Limitations of TEES for MEPs includes the inability to manage disease that extends

Table 2 The modified Fisch–Mattox classification system	
Grade	Definition
A1	Tumor margins completely visible on otoscopy
A2	Tumor margins not completely visible on otoscopy
B1	Tumor filling the middle ear and extending into the hypotympanum or sinus tympani
B2	Tumor filling the middle ear and in the mastoid
B3	Tumor eroding into the carotid canal

From Sanna M, Fois P, Pasanisi E, et al. Middle ear and mastoid glomus tumors (glomus tympanicum): an algorithm for the surgical management. Auris Nasus Larynx 2010;37(6):661–8.

Table 3	
The Glasscock-Jackson classification system	
Grade	**Definition**
1	Tumor margins completely visible on otoscopy
2	Tumor filling the middle ear
3	Tumor filling the middle ear and in the mastoid
4	Tumor extending through the tympanic membrane into the external auditory canal

From Jackson CG, Leonetti JP, Marz SJ. Surgery for benign tumors of the temporal bone. Glasscock-Shambaugh surgery of the ear. 6th edition. In: Gulya AJ, Minor LB, Poe DS, editors. Shelton (CT):People's Medical Publishing House; 2010. p. 729–50.

into the mastoid, and difficulty managing bleeding from the tumor as evidenced by the previously discussed cases.

MIDDLE EAR ADENOMA

Middle ear adenomas (MEAs) are rare, slow-growing neoplasms that are thought to originate in the middle ear mucosa.[15] MEAs are grossly vascular tumors that are well-circumscribed despite having no capsule and contain both epithelial and neuroendocrine features. These tumors typically occur in the fifth decade of life and have no gender predilection. The most common presenting symptom is conductive hearing loss, although otalgia or a sensation of aural fullness is also commonly described. These lesions tend to surround the ossicles without erosion.[16] The overwhelming majority of MEAs do not invade or erode the temporal bone or infiltrate the facial nerve. Otoscopic examination is useful for identifying retrotympanic tumefaction, but it is hard to distinguish MEAs from other temporal bone neoplasms. Temporal bone imaging shows a localized tumor in the middle ear without bone destruction. Differential diagnosis of MEAs includes congenital cholesteatoma, carcinoid tumor, schwannoma, teratoma, meningioma, endolymphatic sac tumor, and paraganglioma of the middle ear.[15]

Surgical removal with immediate or delayed reconstruction of hearing is the preferred treatment modality for MEAs. The traditional surgical approach entails a retroauricular incision with or without a mastoidectomy to access the entire middle ear, including the facial recess. TEES is another approach that can be used to manage

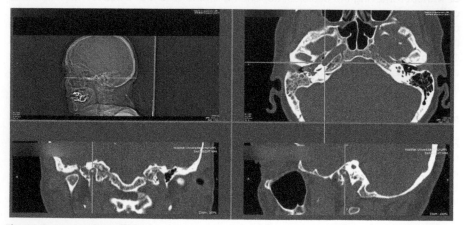

Fig. 1. Image guidance system screen shot showing the middle ear tumor. Note the integrity of the carotid canal.

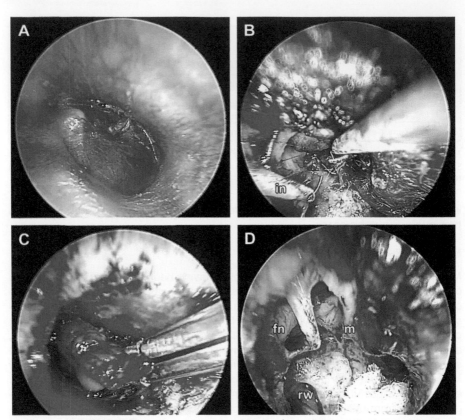

Fig. 2. Edited endoscopic images of a tympanic glomus surgery. The tumor was not embolized. (*A*) Otoscopic view during surgery inspection. (*B*) Dissection of the tumor, finding its point of insertion usually at the area of the Jacobsen nerve. It is important the use of a small bipolar forceps. (*C*) Removal of the tumor. (*D*) inspection of the middle ear cavity after the removal of the tumor. fn, facial nerve; In, incus; m, malleus; rw, round window.

MEAs. Similar to the open approach, complete tumor excision can be performed with or without removing the ossicles, depending on the extent of disease. Marchioni and colleagues[14] reported using TEES to remove 2 MEAs with preservation of the ossicular chain in one of case. The duration of follow-up in this series was less than 1 year and no specific comment was made on recurrence.[14] Local recurrences rates as high as 18% to 22% are reported and typically require revision surgery. Adjuvant radiotherapy or chemotherapy as used for pulmonary or gastrointestinal carcinoid, even when the labyrinth is nonfunctioning, is discouraged.[17]

PETROUS APEX CHOLESTEROL GRANULOMA

PACG is a nonneoplastic, inflammatory, cystic lesion that arises when blood (typically from adjacent bone marrow) fills a mucosa-lined air cell.[18,19] These lesions can occur in any age group and can be discovered incidentally or present with a myriad of symptoms, including headache, double vision, facial anesthesia, facial weakness, hearing loss, and dizziness.[20] There does not seem to be an age, side, or gender predilection for the formation of PACGs.

PACG have a characteristic radiographic appearance on MRI with a hyperintense appearance on T1- and T2-weighted images. Computed tomography often demonstrates a smooth-walled lesion centered with the petrous apex with eroded or absent septations. Effusion, mucocele, chondroid series tumors, chordoma, meningioma, schwannoma, vascular malformations, and epidermoid should all be included in the differential diagnosis of a petrous apex lesion. Asymmetric pneumatization is also a very important consideration in the differential diagnosis because this entity has very similar MRI characteristics to PACG, which can usually be differentiated on high-resolution computed tomography.[20]

Management options for PACG primarily depend on whether the patient is symptomatic and the location of the lesion. Patients with incidentally discovered PACGs or whose symptoms cannot definitively be attributed to the lesion are best managed with observation using serial imaging.[21] Symptomatic patients are best managed with marsupialization, which can be performed via a variety of approaches. Selecting a surgical approach to the petrous apex depends on a number of factors, including the patient's hearing status and the location of the lesion relative to the sphenoid sinus, carotid artery, and jugular bulb.[22,23]

PACGs that are more medially located and adjacent to the sphenoid sinus are excellent candidates for a transnasal approach, where a wide opening can be created that facilitates easy postoperative inspection.[24] The primary advantages of a transnasal approach include no need for an incision, easy postoperative clinical inspection, and the ability to create a wide fenestration into the lesion. Disadvantages of the transnasal approach include the need to remove normal nasal anatomy (turbinates, posterior nasal septum), and the increased level of difficulty in lesions that are more laterally located.[24]

A number of lateral approaches provide access to the petrous apex. The status of the patient's hearing and the location of the PACG are the primary factors when selecting a lateral approach to the petrous apex.[25] Hearing-preserving, otic capsule–sparing approaches include infracochlear, infralabyrinthine, subarcuate, retrolabyrinthine/sinodural angle, middle fossa, and supracochlear.[22] Patient's with long-standing nonserviceable hearing can be managed with a number of nonotic capsule sparing approaches, including the translabyrinthine approach for posterior petrous apex lesions and a transotic or modified transcochlear approach for lesions located in the anterior petrous apex.[20]

An exclusive endoscopic transcanal approach for PACG has not been reported to date. The infracochlear tract has been shown to be easily accessible using a transcanal endoscopic approach (**Fig. 3**). Marchioni and colleagues[3] reported the use on an exclusively endoscopic infracochlear approach to remove cholesteatoma extension into the petrous apex in 3 patients, and to biopsy a chondroma in 1 patient. These authors have each performed an exclusive transcanal endoscopic infracochlear approach for a PACG without complication with limited long-term follow-up for each patient. Advantages of TEES include improved visualization and illumination within the lesion and elimination of the postauricular incision and its attendant opening and closing time. An additional advantage of TEES for the management of PACG is the ability to open loculations that are not within the line of site using angled scopes and instrumentation. Disadvantages of TEES for the management of PACG is potential difficulty in controlling bleeding from the jugular bulb or the carotid artery. A high jugular bulb that closely approximates the first genu of the petrous carotid artery would potentially severely limit the size of the infracochlear opening into a PACG, thus necessitating an alternative approach.[3]

OTHER LESIONS

A number of other temporal bone pathologies managed with a combined microscope open endoscopic approach or an exclusively endoscopic approach have been

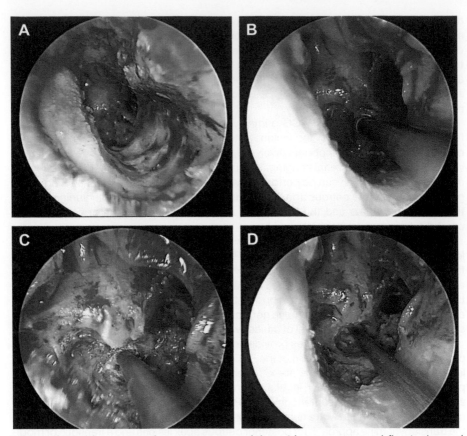

Fig. 3. Infracochlear approach to petrous apex. (*A*) A wide tympanomeatal flap is elevated including exposure of the inferior osseous annulus and hypotympanum. (*B*) The hypotympanic air cells are opened with a drill. (*C*, *D*) The hypotympotomy is extended medially within the boundaries of the petrous carotid artery, jugular bulb, and inferior basal turn of the cochlea.

reported. Marchioni and colleagues[3,14,26] have used TEES alone as well as in combination with an open microscopic approach for removal of intracochlear and intracanalicular schwannomas, a facial nerve hemangioma, cholesteatoma, chondroma, and a geniculate facial hemangioma.

SUMMARY

Middle ear and temporal bone lesions can be removed safely and effectively using TEES, while avoiding mastoid drilling, and a retroauricular incision. TEES provides an unparalleled view of middle ear and medial temporal bone anatomy. In the event that the tympanic membrane and/or the ossicular chain is removed or damaged by the approach of by pathology, reconstruction is possible using TEES. There is a significant learning curve in the adoption of TEES to address tympanic membrane and ossicular pathology that is even more challenging with more complicated pathologic entities affecting the temporal bone.

REFERENCES

1. Tarabichi M. Endoscopic middle ear surgery. Ann Otol Rhinol Laryngol 1999; 108(1):39–46.
2. Tarabichi M, Nogueira JF, Marchioni D, et al. Transcanal endoscopic management of cholesteatoma. Otolaryngol Clin North Am 2013;46(2):107–30.
3. Marchioni D, Alicandri-Ciufelli M, Rubini A, et al. Endoscopic transcanal corridors to the lateral skull base: initial experiences. Laryngoscope 2015;125(Suppl 5): S1–13.
4. Weissman JL, Hirsch BE. Beyond the promontory: the multifocal origin of glomus tympanicum tumors. AJNR Am J Neuroradiol 1998;19(1):119–22.
5. Sweeney AD, Carlson ML, Wanna GB, et al. Glomus tympanicum tumors. Otolaryngol Clin North Am 2015;48(2):293–304.
6. Sennaroglu L, Sungur A. Histopathology of paragangliomas. Otol Neurotol 2002; 23(1):104–5.
7. Schwaber MK, Glasscock ME, Nissen AJ, et al. Diagnosis and management of catecholamine secreting glomus tumors. Laryngoscope 1984;94(8):1008–15.
8. Lee JH, Barich F, Karnell LH, et al. National Cancer Data Base report on malignant paragangliomas of the head and neck. Cancer 2002;94(3):730–7.
9. Boedeker CC, Ridder GJ, Schipper J. Paragangliomas of the head and neck: diagnosis and treatment. Fam Cancer 2005;4(1):55–9.
10. Carlson ML, Sweeney AD, Pelosi S, et al. Glomus tympanicum: a review of 115 cases over 4 decades. Otolaryngol Head Neck Surg 2015;152(1):136–42.
11. Sanna M, Fois P, Pasanisi E, et al. Middle ear and mastoid glomus tumors (glomus tympanicum): an algorithm for the surgical management. Auris Nasus Larynx 2010;37(6):661–8.
12. Jackson C, Leonetti J, Marz S. Surgery for benign tumors of the temporal bone. In: Gulya AJ, Minor LB, Poe D, editors. Glasscock-Shambaugh surgery of the ear. 6th edition. Shelton (CT): People's Medical Publishing House-USA; 2010. p. 729–50.
13. Fisch U. Infratemporal fossa approach for extensive tumors of the temporal bone and base of skull. In: Silverstein H, Norrell HA, editors. Neurological surgery of the ear. Birmingham (AL): Aesculapius Publishing Co; 1977. p. 34–53.
14. Marchioni D, Alicandri-Ciufelli M, Gioacchini FM, et al. Transcanal endoscopic treatment of benign middle ear neoplasms. Eur Arch Otorhinolaryngol 2013; 270(12):2997–3004.
15. Isenring D, Pezier TF, Vrugt B, et al. Middle ear adenoma: case report and discussion. Case Rep Otolaryngol 2014;2014:342125.
16. Pelosi S, Koss S. Adenomatous tumors of the middle ear. Otolaryngol Clin North Am 2015;48(2):305–15.
17. Krouse JH, Nadol JB Jr, Goodman ML. Carcinoid tumors of the middle ear. Ann Otol Rhinol Laryngol 1990;99(7 Pt 1):547–52.
18. Jackler RK, Cho M. A new theory to explain the genesis of petrous apex cholesterol granuloma. Otol Neurotol 2003;24(1):96–106 [discussion: 106].
19. Pfister MH, Jackler RK, Kunda L. Aggressiveness in cholesterol granuloma of the temporal bone may be determined by the vigor of its blood source. Otol Neurotol 2007;28(2):232–5.
20. Isaacson B. Cholesterol granuloma and other petrous apex lesions. Otolaryngol Clin North Am 2015;48(2):361–73.
21. Sweeney AD, Osetinsky LM, Carlson ML, et al. The natural history and management of petrous apex cholesterol granulomas. Otol Neurotol 2015;36(10):1714–9.

22. Isaacson B, Kutz JW, Roland PS. Lesions of the petrous apex: diagnosis and management. Otolaryngol Clin North Am 2007;40(3):479–519, viii.
23. Isaacson B, Kutz JW Jr, Mendelsohn D, et al. CT venography: use in selecting a surgical approach for the treatment of petrous apex cholesterol granulomas. Otol Neurotol 2009;30(3):386–91.
24. Zanation AM, Snyderman CH, Carrau RL, et al. Endoscopic endonasal surgery for petrous apex lesions. Laryngoscope 2009;119(1):19–25.
25. Rihani J, Kutz JW Jr, Isaacson B. Hearing outcomes after surgical drainage of petrous apex cholesterol granuloma. J Neurol Surg B Skull Base 2015;76(3): 171–5.
26. Marchioni D, Soloperto D, Genovese E, et al. Facial nerve hemangioma of the geniculate ganglion: an endoscopic surgical approach. Auris Nasus Larynx 2014;41(6):576–81.

Outcomes Following Endoscopic Stapes Surgery

Jacob B. Hunter, MD, Alejandro Rivas, MD*

KEYWORDS

- Endoscopic • Stapes • Stapedotomy • Stapedectomy • Outcomes
- Endoscopic ear surgery

KEY POINTS

- With experience, endoscopic stapes surgery is an effective alternative when compared to microscopic stapes surgery, with similar complication rates and audiometric outcomes.
- To date, 56.0% to 86.7% patients have had closure of their air bone gaps to under 10 dB HL following endoscopic stapes surgeries.
- Postoperative dysgeusia and pain scores appear to be improved in endoscopic stapes surgeries compared with microscopic approaches.

 Video content accompanies this article at http://www.oto.theclinics.com.

INTRODUCTION

The first published case of use of an endoscope in the middle ear was in 1967, when it was used to visualize the middle ear and the integrity of the ossicular chain through a myringotomy incision.[1] With technological improvements leading to enhanced image resolution, as well as recognized acceptance of endoscopes within the field of rhinology, there has been greater implementation of endoscopes in otologic and neurotologic procedures. Now, almost 50 years after the first endoscopic description of the middle ear, surgeons are utilizing endoscopes to evaluate and remove cholesteatomas,[2–4] place cochlear implants,[5] remove vestibular schwannomas,[6] and assist with repairing dehiscent superior semicircular canals.[7] Although many of these applications are limited to a few scattered case reports, several endoscopic cholesteatoma studies have highlighted the role endoscopes play in identifying residual disease. Given the endoscope's wide angle of view and improved visualization of structures parallel to the microscope,[8] it is not surprising that there are several reports describing the role of endoscopes in stapes procedures. This article provides a summary of

Department of Otolaryngology-Head and Neck Surgery, Vanderbilt University Medical Center, 1215 21st Avenue South, Suite 7209, Nashville, TN 37232, USA
* Corresponding author.
E-mail address: alejandro.rivas@vanderbilt.edu

Otolaryngol Clin N Am 49 (2016) 1215–1225
http://dx.doi.org/10.1016/j.otc.2016.05.012
0030-6665/16/$ – see front matter © 2016 Elsevier Inc. All rights reserved.

endoscopic stapes surgery, highlighting the variety of techniques and perceived advantages, as well as audiometric and patient outcomes (**Fig. 1**).

SURGICAL TECHNIQUE

An endoscopic stapedotomy or stapedectomy is essentially the same technical procedure as with a microscope, but a few subtle differences do exist. Although some surgeons infiltrate the ear canal with 2% lidocaine in 1:100,000 epinephrine or 0.25% Marcaine in 1:200,000 epinephrine, others place cotton balls soaked in 1:2000 or 1:5000 epinephrine for approximately 5 minutes.[9] Regardless of the technique, hemostasis is paramount to all endoscopic ear surgery, with the surgeon

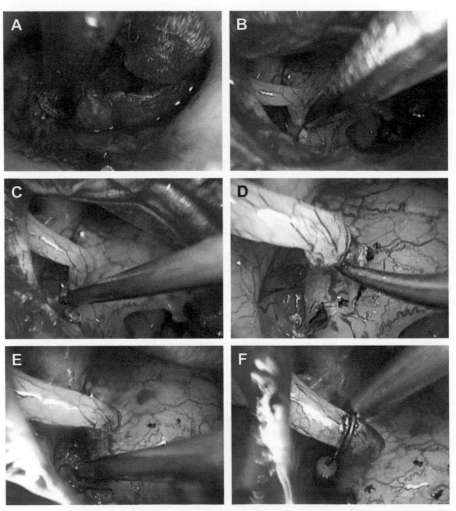

Fig. 1. Panels A–F demonstrate the various steps of a stapedotomy, while highlighting the visualization obtained with an endoscope. (*A*) Elevating the flap, in this case, utilizing a custom suction elevator. (*B*) Sectioning the stapedial tendon, in this case, with microscissors. (*C*) Lasering the posterior stapes crus. (*D*) Downfracturing the stapes superstructure. (*E*) Lasering the footplate to create a fenestra. (*F*) Utilizing the laser to crimp a Nitinol prosthesis.

unable to suction during dissection since his or her nondominant hand is typically holding the endoscope. The ear canal skin is then incised approximately 5 to 8 mm lateral to the posterior annulus, allowing elevation of a tympanomeatal flap, and providing access to the middle ear space. With a 0° or 30° endoscope, the incudos-tapedial joint and oval window niche can almost always be visualized; however, occasionally a variable amount of scutum still needs to be removed to allow instrument access to the region. Once stapes fixation is confirmed, and adequate exposure is obtained, the stapedial tendon is divided. Depending on the surgeon or institution, lasers or microdrills are used to divide the anterior or posterior stapes crus. If one is performing a laser stapedioplasty, the laser is then used to create a small gap in the footplate, posterior to the otosclerotic focus, enabling removal of the otospongiosis involved footplate and crura. In a stapedotomy, a laser, typically CO_2 or potassium titanyl phosphate (KTP), or microdrill, creates a fenestra in the footplate, followed by placement of a piston-type prosthesis. If a stapedectomy is undertaken, tragal perichondrium is typically harvested and used to cover the oval window, followed by placement of the prosthesis between the lenticular process of the incus and the oval window. The tympanomeatal flap is returned to position, and depending on the surgeon, absorbable packing is placed in the ear canal.

INTRAOPERATIVE ISSUES

Several intraoperative issues have been identified since the first endoscopic stapes procedure was described by Tarabichi in 1999[8] (**Box 1**). Although the report described 165 middle ear surgeries that the primary author performed solely with the endoscope over a 5-year period, 13 of those were stapedectomies.[8] Without reporting significant intraoperative details, the author noted that the endoscope reduced the need for curetting the medial bony canal in order to provide exposure to the oval window niche.[8]

One year later, Poe[10] described using an endoscope adjunctively in performing laser stapedioplasties, designing an endoscope with a 200-μm diameter argon laser fiber protruding from the distal tip. The laser was then used to lyse the anterior crus, followed by a row of overlapping burns on the footplate, allowing separation of the footplate between the anterior and middle thirds.[10] No specific intraoperative issues were addressed, and the remainder of the procedure was performed using the microscope.

In 2011, Nogueira and colleagues[9] reported on their experience with endoscopic stapedotomies, addressing perceived differences between microscopic and endoscopic approaches to stapes surgery. Noting that the microscope is limited by direct line of sight during procedures, while endoscopes allow the surgeon to look around corners, the authors assessed 15 patients undergoing endoscopic stapedotomies and reported that the oval window niche, the tympanic segment of the facial nerve, and pyramidal process were all able to be visualized with a 0° endoscope in 8 patients

---

Box 1
Intraoperative issues

Improved visualization

Reduced need for curretting medial bony canal

Decreased chorda tympani manipulation

Difficulty manipulating microdrill with the endoscope

Reduced patient head positioning

(53.3%).[9] However, when utilizing a 30° endoscope, the same structures were all visualized in 12 patients (80%).[9] In regards to the chorda tympani nerve, they reported that only 3 patients (20%) required manipulation of the nerve to complete the procedure, implying that endoscopes lead to decreased chorda tympani nerve handling compared with microscope cases.[9] Evaluating their ability to perform the procedure, the anterior crus was fractured in all cases with the 30° endoscope, and although there was some difficulty in placing the prosthesis, no intraoperative complications were reported.[9] This highlights an important issue within all endoscopic ear surgery, since although endoscopes provide improved visualization of middle ear structures, commonly used instruments may not be able to access every location visualized.

Despite the limitation, and many surgeons' concern regarding the need for new instrumentation and monitors to perform endoscopic ear surgery, Nogueira and colleagues[9] purposely worked with endoscopes and microinstruments that most hospitals in which otolaryngologic procedures are performed would have available. And despite use of sinus endoscopes, Nogueira and colleagues[9] emphasized that longer endoscopes do not interfere with the hand movement by remaining in different horizontal planes.

In 2012, Sarkar and colleagues[11] reported their endoscopic stapedotomy results in 30 patients, using 0° and 45° pediatric nasal endoscopes, with a diameter of 2.7 mm, utilizing conventional ear surgery instruments. They found that there was significant difficulty in manipulating the drill and the endoscope within the ear canal; thus they completed all bone removal with a curette.[11] Of interest, prior to performing the surgeries, the authors originally tried using 4 mm and 18 cm long endoscopes on cadavers, but with operational difficulty, they attempted to use 1.9 mm diameter endoscopes.[11] However, limited by poor illumination with the smaller endoscopes, they eventually used pediatric nasal endoscopes to perform the surgeries.[11]

Migirov and Wolf[12] presented their endoscopic stapedotomy technique in 2013, reporting preliminary results on 8 consecutive patients, with at least 6 months of follow-up. All surgeries were performed with a 0° endoscope, although a 30° endoscope was utilized to obtain better visualization of the oval window niche, the anterior crus of the stapes, the tympanic facial nerve segment, and pyramidal eminence in 2 cases due to excessive bony overhang of the medial bony canal.[12] This allowed them to avoid any curettage or drilling of the scutum, as well as avoiding chorda tympani nerve mobilization, while creating the footplate fenestra with a curved 0.5 mm diameter diamond burr.[12] Noting the physical limitations of the scutum, the authors commented on the improved comfort of a right-handed surgeon performing surgery on right ears, with the relative difficultly in left ears in fenestrating the footplate and positioning the prosthesis.[12] With their experience, the authors suggested that the endoscopic approach should be utilized in patients with unfavorable external or middle ear anatomy, those with food-, smell- or taste-related occupations, revision or bilateral stapedotomy candidates, those with already impaired taste sensation, and in those for whom the taste of food contributes to their quality of life.[12]

In 2014, Kojima and colleagues[13] compared 15 patients who underwent endoscopic stapes surgery, with an average follow-up of 8.6 months, against 35 patients and 41 ears who had microscopic stapes surgery and an average follow-up of 27.2 months. Noting that Japanese patients tend to have narrow and curved external auditory canals, in Japan, stapes surgery is routinely performed via a posterior or anterior auricular incision. Thus with unfavorable external ear anatomy for the direct line of sight with the microscope, the authors utilized 2.7 and 4 mm wide, 18 cm long, 0° endoscopes, routinely drilling the bony wall in the posterosuperior part of the canal until the pyramidal eminence and tympanic segment of the facial nerve were visualized.[13]

Following prosthesis placement, gelfoam was placed around the footplate fenestra to prevent perilymphatic fistula formation.[13] Assessing the length of the procedure between procedural types, they found no significant difference in time, 54.1 minutes in the endoscopic group versus 53.0 minutes in the microscopic group.[13] The authors noted that when the extent of drilling was adequate for endoscopic surgery, providing visualization of the facial nerve, only the area around the incudostapedial joint could be clearly seen with the microscope.[13]

In 2015, Daneshi and Jahnadideh[14] described their endoscopic stapedotomy experience, highlighting their practice in using no postoperative packing in hopes of minimizing patient annoyance. In regards to their technique, following prosthesis placement, no absorbable materials were placed in the middle ear, and the tympano-meatal flap was repositioned and fixed with tissue adhesive.[14] They performed 19 endoscopic stapedotomies, comparing them with a control group of 15 microscopic stapedotomies; all patients were questioned approximately 6 hours postoperatively about the degree of satisfaction using a visual analog scale.[14] In the endoscopic cohort, utilizing 0° and 30° degree endoscopes, they noted that in 7 (36.8%) cases, no bony removal was required for visualization and access to the oval window niche, while six (31.6%) patients did require minimal curettage, and the chorda tympani nerve was preserved in all cases.[14] Given the reduced need for bony removal, the surgical time was significantly shorter in the endoscopic group as compared with the conventional group, 31.8 minutes as opposed to 54.3 minutes ($P<.05$).[14] The authors postulated that reduced patient positioning, as well as less dissection and maneuvers, may partially explain the reduced time in the endoscopic group compared with the microscopic group.[14] However, the authors do not mention how the procedures were timed. The authors posit that endoscopic stapes surgery reduces the need for turning the head in difficult situations, such as those patients with obese short necks, or patients with cervical osteoarthritis.[14]

Marchioni and colleagues[15] recently published their exclusive endoscopic management of stapes malformations in 17 patients, 6 of whom underwent either a stapedotomy or stapedectomy depending on the intraoperative findings. Of the 6 patients, 1 patient had a low intraoperative gusher, controlled with positioning the prosthesis, bovine perichondrium, and fibrin glue, with complete preservation of hearing and closure of the air–bone gap to 5 dB.[15] In 2 other patients, 1 patient had a monopodalic stapes, fused with the footplate, requiring a stapedectomy, while another had a persistent stapedial artery, allowing them to create a stapedotomy anterior to the artery.[15] However, the authors did not comment on the advantages or disadvantages of using the endoscope in their patient population. Nonetheless, the authors believe that the use of endoscopes in challenging anatomy cases, such as malformations and revision cases (**Fig. 2**), is advantageous, while also recognizing that deep oval window niches are better suited to microscopic stapedotomies given the lack of depth perception during endoscopic procedures.

Hunter and colleagues[16] recently reported on a multicenter experience, consisting of 68 subjects who underwent endoscopic stapes surgery over approximately a 5-year period between 4 tertiary otologic referral centers. Although 18 patients were excluded from the data analysis, the authors provided preliminary analysis regarding surgical technique with several surgeons utilizing either a 0° or 30° endoscope. They specifically noted that scutum anatomy prevented prosthesis placement with a straight and curved alligator in 77.1% and 67.3% of cases, respectively. Furthermore, 94.0% of cases required manipulation of the chorda tympani nerve, leading to nerve transection in 12.0% of patients. Intraoperatively, 8.0% of patients had tympanic membrane perforations that were repaired with a perichondrium graft; 4.0% of

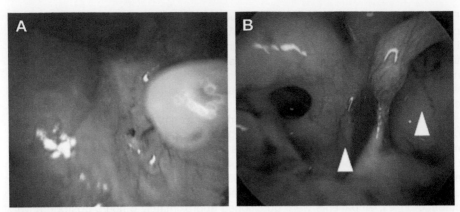

Fig. 2. (*A*) The image is of revision case in which the patient had persistent conductive hearing loss following stapedectomy, with the endoscope enabling improved visualization of the oval window niche, and appreciation that the wire hook was too short. (*B*) The image is of a bifid facial nerve (*arrowheads*).

patients had floating footplates, and 2.0% of patients had incus subluxation. Between all 4 centers, the average operative time was 77.4 minutes (35–170 minutes). Although no reference or comparison was made to a microscopic population, the authors believe their results reinforce the safety of endoscopic stapes surgery, while also highlighting the variety of reports describing removal of the bony medial external canal wall, not for visualization, but for manipulation of the stapes and stapes prosthesis (Video 1).

Audiologic Outcomes

There is no standard in reporting audiometric outcomes following endoscopic stapes surgeries, let alone microscopic stapes surgeries in general. Nonetheless, the few endoscopic reports allow for a simple comparison, as outlined in **Table 1**. In Tarabichi's initial report, postoperatively, only 7 patients had at least 1-year of follow-up, with 6 patients having a postoperative air–bone gap (pure tone average of 0.5, 1, and 2 kHz) under 10 dB HL.[8] The author defined postoperative sensorineural hearing loss as greater than a 10 dB HL change in bone conduction average at 0.5, 1, 2, and 3 kHz, reporting that no patients had sensorineural hearing loss postoperatively.[8]

Although Poe[10] reported on 34 patients who underwent stapes surgeries, 11 of whom had a stapedioplasty as previously described, only 5 were completed the laser endoscope. Although individual patient audiometric data were reported, those patients who underwent the procedure with the laser endoscope were unable to be identified from the report's tables.

Nogueira and colleagues[9] did not report individual audiometric data, but stated that all patients had subjective improvement in their hearing at postoperative day 15, with 14 patients (93.3%) having audiogram improvements. Summarizing all 15 patients, the mean preoperative speech reception threshold was 65 dB HL, which improved to 25 dB HL postoperatively.[9]

Sarkar and colleagues[11] reported that the mean preoperative air–bone gap was 41.5 plus or minus 5.2 dB HL, improving to 10.1 plus or minus 3.6 dB HL 3 months postoperatively, which was statistically significant. They further described that 93% of patients had closure of their air–bone gap to 15 dB HL or less.[11] By comparing the preoperative and postoperative bone conduction pure tone average (0.5, 1, 2,

Table 1
Tabulated patient outcomes

Author, Year	N	Procedure	Follow-up (mo)	Audiometric Outcomes	Chorda Tympani Comments	Surgical Time
Tarabichi,[8] 1999	13	Stapedectomy	≥12	ABG <10 dB 85.7%	N/A	N/A
Poe,[10] 2000	5	Stapedioplasty	N/A	N/A	N/A	N/A
Marchioni et al,[15] 2015	6	Stapedectomy and stapedotomy	N/A	ABG <10 dB 83.3%, 100.0% <20 dB	N/A	N/A
Nogueira et al,[9] 2011	15	Stapedotomy	1–1.3	ABG <25 dB 93.3%	Manipulated in 20.0%	N/A
Migirov & Wolf,[12] 2013	8	Stapedotomy	≥6	ABG <10 dB 75.0%, 100.0% <20 dB	100.0% preservation rate	N/A
Sarkar,[11] 2013	30	Stapedotomy	3	ABG <10 dB 56.0%, 100.0% <20 dB	N/A	N/A
Daneshi & Jahandideh,[14] 2016	19	Stapedotomy	N/A	ABG <10 dB 57.9%, 93.7% <20 dB	100.0% preservation rate	31.8
Kojima et al,[13] 2014	15	Stapedotomy	8.6	ABG <10 dB 86.7%, 93.3% <20 dB	No postoperative dysgeusia	53.0
Hunter,[16] 2015	50	Stapedectomy and stapedotomy	13.4	ABG <20 dB 90.0%	88.0% preservation rate	77.4

and 4 kHz) to assess for sensorineural hearing loss, the average change was only 0.1 plus or minus 0.7 dB HL, with 80% of patients demonstrating bone conduction improvements following the procedure.[11]

Migirov and Wolf[12] reported the preoperative average air conduction threshold (0.5, 1.0, and 2 kHz) in their patient sample was 64 dB HL, which improved to 30.6 dB HL postoperatively. Demonstrating no sensorineural hearing loss, the mean preoperative bone conduction thresholds, at the same frequencies, were 29.8 dB HL, improving to 25.1 dB HL postoperatively.[12] When the mean preoperative air–bone gap was 31.4 dB HL, 6 patients had closure to under 10 dB HL following the procedure, while the remaining 2 patients were between 10 and 15 dB HL.[12]

Kojima and colleagues[13] assessed hearing 2 to 7 months postoperatively in the endoscopic group and 6 to 12 months in the microscopic group. In the endoscopic group, 86.7% of ears had closure of their postoperative air–bone gap to 10 dB HL or less, while 1 patient each had postoperative air–bone gaps between 11 and 20 dB HL and 21 and 30 dB HL.[13]

Daneshi and Jahnadideh,[14] at an average follow-up of 7.4 months, noted that 11 patients (57.9%) had a postoperative air–bone gap between 0 and 10 dB HL, while 18 patients (94.7%) had a postoperative air–bone gap between 0 and 20 dB HL, and no patient suffered from profound hearing loss postoperatively.

Although the Marchioni and colleagues[15] hearing data should be interpreted with caution, since only malformed stapes operations were reported, in those patients either undergoing a stapedotomy or stapedectomy, the preoperative mean bone conduction threshold and air–bone gaps were 25.4 dB HL and 36.3 dB HL, respectively. Postoperatively, the mean bone conduction threshold and air–bone gaps were 25.6 dB HL and 7.8 dB HL, respectively.[15] Although complications were not broken down individually, of the 17 patients reported, no postoperative complications were documented, and all patients were discharged on postoperative day 1.[15]

In the authors' experience, with an average follow-up of 13.4 months (0.76–57.4 months), the average postoperative air–bone gap was 11.2 dB HL, a statistically significant improvement compared with the preoperative mean of 33.1 dB HL ($P<.001$). When the authors compared surgical techniques, noting 3 different techniques were utilized between 4 different institutions, endoscopic laser stapedotomy, endoscopic drill stapedotomy, and endoscopic laser stapedectomy, all 3 techniques demonstrated significant improvements in pure tone averages and air–bone gaps postoperatively, although no statistical significance was noted between groups. Assessing all subjects, 90.0% of patients had their air–bone gap closed to under 20 dB HL, although 2 patients had greater than a 30 dB HL sensorineural hearing loss following the procedure. Because both patients were from institutions that did not have access to lasers, the authors hypothesized that the sensorineural hearing loss was the result of drilling on the stapes crura and footplate. They further believe that the lack of depth perception when using endoscopes may affect outcomes using a microdrill. However, the authors believe improved outcomes might result from using the laser to create the fenestra in an endoscopic stapedotomy. When those patients who did not have access to lasers because of institutional differences were removed for data analysis, no patient had sensorineural hearing loss, and 88.2% of patients had air–bone gap closures under 15 dB HL.

In summary, from all available reports, a range of 56.0% to 86.7% of patients had closure of their air–bone gaps under 10 dB HL. When assessing those patients who had postoperative air–bone gaps under 20 dB HL, no study reported a rate worse than 90.0%. Although 2 patients, amounting to 1.2% of all reported endoscopic stapes procedures, had sensorineural hearing loss, it was hypothesized to be secondary to use of the drill on the stapes crura and footplate. This highlights the importance of using the laser as an ideal adjuvant tool when working on the footplate.

Patient Outcomes

To date, there are few reported outcomes following endoscopic stapes surgeries. Nogueira and colleagues[9] noted that postoperatively, 1 patient complained of a reduction in taste, which resolved in 15 days. In addition, although no tympanic membrane perforations or canal hematomas were noted, 1 patient had postoperative vertigo, treated with medicine, which resolved by postoperative day 15.[9]

Migirov and Wolf[12] reported that all 8 of their patients described their postoperative taste function as normal. Recognizing that many countries will admit patients postoperatively, and many institutions in the United States discharge the same day following the procedure, per institutional norms, all but 1 patient was discharged 2 days after surgery, while the remaining patient developed vertigo on postoperative day 1, treated with intravenous amoxicillin clavulanate and steroids. The patient's symptoms resolved 1 week following surgery.[12]

Despite the reporting of standard stapes surgery postoperative complications, Kojima and colleagues[13] were the first study to assess postoperative outcomes utilizing a simple questionnaire. Each endoscopic patient was questioned about the severity of pain approximately 6 hours following surgery.[13] The severity was recorded using 3 options: almost no pain, mild pain requiring no analgesics, and pain requiring analgesics.[13] When asked about the severity of postoperative pain, 93.3% of patients reported either "almost no pain" or "mild pain requiring no analgesics."[13] Of note, 4 patients underwent bilateral procedures, wherein a microscopic technique was used on 1 ear, and an endoscopic technique was used on the contralateral ear. All patients reported that they suffered from "irritating pain for 2 to 3 days" following the microscopic approach, but had no pain following the endoscopic surgery.[13]

When Kojima and colleagues[13] assessed their postoperative complications, 1 patient developed late facial paralysis 10 days postoperatively, which resolved within 1 month. In the endoscopic group, no patient developed postoperative dysgeusia, while in the microscopic group, transient abnormal taste sensation, presumably caused by intraoperative chorda tympani traction, occurred in 4 patients (11.4%).[13] Postoperative dizziness was mild in all patients who received endoscopic surgery, with 12 (80.0%) patients reporting dizziness for 1 day, compared with 25 (71.4%) patients in the microscopic group.[13]

Similar to Kojima and colleagues, Daneshi and Jahnadideh[14] also assessed postoperative patient satisfaction, utilizing a visual analog scale that consisted of a 100 mm horizontal line, with the 2 ends representing extremes of satisfaction and dissatisfaction. They reported that the endoscopic group indicated higher satisfaction compared with the microscopic group, 78.8 versus 62.9 mm ($P < .05$). No patient had facial nerve paralysis or intraoperative chorda tympani nerve transections, while 2 patients complained of postoperative transient vertigo.[14]

The authors recently reported that postoperatively, 10.0% of subjects complained of altered taste; 4.0% required a short course of systemic steroids for dizziness that resolved after 10 days, and 1 subject each was noted to have an extruded prosthesis, mild otitis externa, and a posterosuperior tympanic membrane retraction at last follow-up.

Summarizing outcomes, although no permanent facial nerve injuries have occurred, and the incidence of postoperative dizziness is comparable to microscopic procedures, postoperative dysgeusia and pain scores appear to be improved in endoscopic stapes surgeries compared with microscopic approaches. Nonetheless, with only 161 reported endoscopic stapes cases to date, further prospective studies with larger patient populations are warranted.

SUMMARY

Despite the few reports to date, endoscopic stapes surgery is an effective alternative compared with microscopic stapes surgery, with similar complication rates and audiometric outcomes. Future studies effectively assessing the influence of 30° endoscopes and the perceived reduced need for bony removal, as well as patient-centered outcomes, are warranted. Although studies suggest that endoscopes provide improved visualization of the footplate given the overall reported reduced need of scutum removal, future studies are needed assess not only improved visualization, but instrumentation access to the oval window. And while the authors believe visualization advantages make endoscopes ideally suited for revision and malformed stapes, further data and outcomes are needed. Some authors suggest the cost-effectiveness of endoscopic surgery could be an important factor in developing countries, without supplying data,[11] while most agree that the endoscopy allows appropriate evaluation of ossicular anatomy, articulation, and mobility.[15]

SUPPLEMENTARY DATA

Supplementary data related to this article can be found at http://dx.doi.org/10.1016/j.otc.2016.05.012.

REFERENCES

1. Mer SB, Derbyshire AJ, Brushenko A, et al. Fiberoptic endotoscopes for examining the middle ear. Arch Otolaryngol 1967;85(4):387–93.
2. McKennan KX. Endoscopic 'second look' mastoidoscopy to rule out residual epitympanic/mastoid cholesteatoma. Laryngoscope 1993;103(7):810–4.
3. Thomassin JM, Korchia D, Duchon-Doris JM. Residual cholesteatoma: its prevention by surgery with endoscopic guidance. Rev Laryngol Otol Rhinol (Bord) 1991; 112(5):405–8 [in French].
4. Tarabichi M. Endoscopic management of acquired cholesteatoma. Am J Otol 1997;18(5):544–9.
5. Dia A, Nogueira JF, O'Grady KM, et al. Report of endoscopic cochlear implantation. Otol Neurotol 2014;35(10):1755–8.
6. Setty P, D'Andrea KP, Stucken EZ, et al. Endoscopic resection of vestibular schwannomas. J Neurol Surg B Skull Base 2015;76(3):230–8.
7. Carter MS, Lookabaugh S, Lee DJ. Endoscopic-assisted repair of superior canal dehiscence syndrome. Laryngoscope 2014;124(6):1464–8.
8. Tarabichi M. Endoscopic middle ear surgery. Ann Otol Rhinol Laryngol 1999; 108(1):39–46.
9. Nogueira Junior JF, Martins MJ, Aguiar CV, et al. Fully endoscopic stapes surgery (stapedotomy): technique and preliminary results. Braz J Otorhinolaryngol 2011; 77(6):721–7.
10. Poe DS. Laser-assisted endoscopic stapedectomy: a prospective study. Laryngoscope 2000;110(5 Pt 2 Suppl 95):1–37.
11. Sarkar S, Banerjee S, Chakravarty S, et al. Endoscopic stapes surgery: our experience in thirty two patients. Clin Otolaryngol 2013;38(2):157–60.
12. Migirov L, Wolf M. Endoscopic transcanal stapedotomy: how I do it. Eur Arch Otorhinolaryngol 2013;270(4):1547–9.

13. Kojima H, Komori M, Chikazawa S, et al. Comparison between endoscopic and microscopic stapes surgery. Laryngoscope 2014;124(1):266–71.
14. Daneshi A, Jahandideh H. Totally endoscopic stapes surgery without packing: novel technique bringing most comfort to the patients. Eur Arch Otorhinolaryngol 2016;273(3):631–4.
15. Marchioni D, Soloperto D, Villari D, et al. Stapes malformations: the contribute of the endoscopy for diagnosis and surgery. Eur Arch Otorhinolaryngol 2016;273(7): 1723–9.
16. Hunter JB, Zuniga MG, Leite J, et al. Surgical and Audiological Outcomes in Endoscopic Stapes Surgeries Across Four Institutions. Otolaryngology-Head and Neck Surgery 2016;154(6):1093–8.

The Fully Endoscopic Acoustic Neuroma Surgery

Daniele Marchioni, MD[a], Marco Carner, MD[a], Alessia Rubini, MD[a,*],
João Flávio Nogueira, MD[b], Barbara Masotto, MD[c],
Matteo Alicandri-Ciufelli, MD, FEBORL-HNS[d,e], Livio Presutti, MD[d]

KEYWORDS

- Transcanal/Transpromontorial endoscopic approach • Acoustic neuroma
- Facial nerve • Internal auditory canal

KEY POINTS

- Transcanal/transpromontorial endoscopic approach is an effective surgical technique for small intracanalicular acoustic neuroma removal.
- The surgical approach must follow strict landmarks to identify and preserve facial nerve.
- Although there is no possibility for hearing preservation, facial nerve results are encouraging.
- Transcanal/transpromontorial endoscopic approach can be an alternative to wait and scan policy or radiosurgery in this kind of pathology.

INTRODUCTION

Fully endoscopic surgery is a surgical standard of care in minimally invasive neurosurgery of the anterior skull base. The successful implementation of the endoscope in pituitary surgery has allowed many surgeons to adopt the benefits of endoscopy such as panoramic view, brilliant illumination, and faster postoperative recovery. Endoscope use in other areas of the brain, such as the cerebellopontine angle (CPA) and the internal acoustic canal (IAC), however, has been limited.

At present, endoscopy in CPA surgery is primarily used as an adjunct to conventional microscopic surgical techniques, so called endoscope-assisted microsurgery

The authors have nothing to disclose.
[a] Otolaryngology Department, University Hospital of Verona, Borgo Trento Via Aristide Stefani 1, Verona 37100, Italy; [b] Sinus & Oto Centro, Hospital Geral de Fortaleza, Rua Dr. José Furtado 1480, Fortaleza 60822-300, Brazil; [c] Neurosurgery Department, University Hospital of Verona, Borgo Trento Via Aristide Stefani 1, 10, Verona 37100, Italy; [d] Otolaryngology Department, University Hospital of Modena, Via del Pozzo 71, Modena 41100, Italy; [e] Neurosurgery Department, New Civil Hospital Sant'Agostino-Estense, Stradello Baggiovara 53, Baggiovara, MO 41126, Italy
* Corresponding author.
E-mail address: rubinialessia@gmail.com

Otolaryngol Clin N Am 49 (2016) 1227–1236
http://dx.doi.org/10.1016/j.otc.2016.05.014
0030-6665/16/$ – see front matter © 2016 Elsevier Inc. All rights reserved.

(EAM) for removal of acoustic neuromas (ANs). The first introduction of the endoscopic technique in IAC surgery has been in combination with the retrosigmoid approach after removal of the CPA extension of the tumor.

The intracanalicular extension would be removed under endoscopic control, trying to avoid extensive drilling of the posterior aspect of the petrous bone.[1] More recently, a keyhole retrosigmoid approach has been proposed for surgical removal of ANs.[2]

EAM in CPA has been an excellent start for the use of the endoscope in the posterior fossa[3] and the advances in the application of endoscopy in the surgical treatment of middle ear cholesteatoma[4–6] with the natural evolution of the otologic/endoscopic techniques allowed the use of the endoscopes in lateral skull base surgery.

By studying and understanding the endoscopic anatomy and procedures, approaches of the middle ear have been gradually completed until endoscopic anatomy of the labyrinth and IAC were thoroughly known.[7] Recently, a progression from EAM to a fully appropriate endoscopic technique in the internal auditory canal (IAC) surgery has been recorded and applied clinically[8,9] for removal of AN in the IAC.

Retrosigmoid, transmastoid-translabyrinthine, and middle cranial fossa approaches are the most popular surgical approaches to treat pathology extending into the IAC, such as ANs.[10]

All these approaches are characterized by the fact that they are indirect approaches to the inner ear and require wide external incisions and a variable degree of temporal bone removal to access the IAC and CPA.

Hence, the technique outlined in this publication provides a safe and effective step-by-step way to perform CPA surgery using a fully endoscopic transcanal technique for the resection of ANs, as it has superior visualization of the neurovascular relationship allowing for successful resection of ANs.

TRANSCANAL TRANSPROMONTORIAL ENDOSCOPIC APPROACH TO THE INTERNAL AUDITORY CANAL

The transcanal transpromontorial endoscopic approach (TTEA) representing the first fully endoscopic approach for the acoustic neuroma, the external auditory canal (EAC) is used as a natural surgical corridor to reach the fundus of the IAC; passing through the cochlea and the vestibule, exposing the whole IAC from the external auditory canal (**Fig. 1**). From an anatomic point of view, this approach allows work on the medial wall of the tympanic cavity and lateral skull base dissecting the whole IAC from the fundus to the

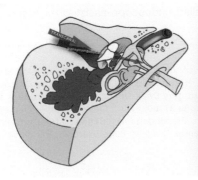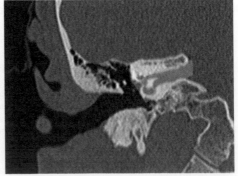

Fig. 1. Schematic drawing on the left representing the surgical corridors; the EAC is used as natural corridors so as to reach the IAC: on the right, a computed tomography scan in coronal view showing in yellow the working area.

porus, avoiding cerebellum, middle and posterior fossa manipulation, reducing the mobility related to the standard procedures (middle cranial fossa, translabyrinthine, and retrosigmoid approaches). However, because cochlea removal is mandatory to have access to the IAC, the sacrifice of hearing function is required (**Fig. 2**).

Indications

We considered indications for this surgical route:

- Acoustic neuroma limited to the IAC growing or symptomatic with hearing loss (type D hearing according to American Academy of Otolaryngology – Head and Neck Surgery [AAO-HNS] classification).
- Cochlear schwannoma with or without IAC involvement.
- Residual acoustic neuroma into the IAC after previous surgery.

Surgical Technique

During surgery, 0° rigid endoscopes (Karl Storz, Tuttlingen, Germany) are used, 15 cm in length and 3 mm or 4 mm in diameter. An AIDA 3-chip high-resolution monitor and camera (Karl Storz) are used.

The patient is in a supine position, the head gently rotated in the contralateral side, and facial nerve monitoring is used (nerve integrity monitor).

A circumferential incision of the skin of the EAC is made with a round knife using the 0° endoscopic view, between the cartilaginous and bony portions of the EAC; the skin is elevated with the eardrum circumferentially detaching the annulus from the bony ring, and the flap, pedicled on the umbus, is transposed laterally and then detached from the malleus using a microscissors. The skin of the EAC with the eardrum is so removal exposing the tympanic cavity and the bony portion of the EAC (**Fig. 3**A).

To gain optimal surgical access to the entire medial wall of the tympanic cavity, the EAC is drilled (**Fig. 3**B) detecting anteriorly the temporomandibular joint, posteriorly the mastoid segment of the facial nerve; the bony annulus is also drilled

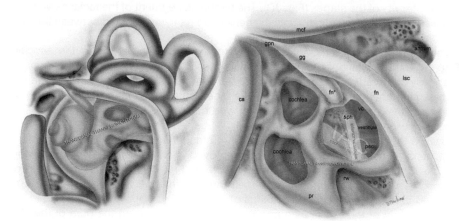

Fig. 2. Left ear; Anatomic landmarks of the transpromontorial transcanal endoscopic approach: the reader can note the position of the facial nerve into the fundus of the IAC and the close relationships among the vestibule, the cochlea, and the IAC. ca, carotid artery; fn*, labyrinthine portion of facial nerve; fn, facial nerve; gg, geniculate ganglion; gpn, greater petrosal nerve; lsc, lateral semicircular canal; mcf, middle cranial fossa; pr, promontory; psc, posterior semicircular canal opening; rw, round window; sph, spherical recess; vc, vestibular crest.

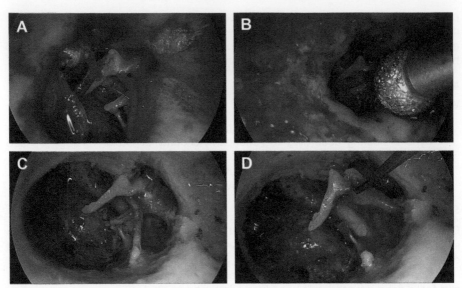

Fig. 3. Left ear; TTEA: (*A*) the eardrum is removed; (*B*) a diamond bur is used to enlarge the EAC; (*C*) after the calibration of the EAC, the tympanic cavity is under endoscopic control; (*D*) ossicular chain removal.

circumferentially exposing the hypotympanum, protympanum, retrotympanum, and attic spaces. After this procedure, good control of the whole tympanic cavity is achieved, and the ossicular chain and promontory region are easily exposed endoscopically (**Fig. 3**C).

The ossicular chain removal is a crucial procedure so as to have good access to the medial whole of the tympanic cavity; the incus and the malleus are removed, maintaining the integrity of the stapes (**Fig. 3**D). The tympanic segment of the facial nerve is so exposed from the second genu until the geniculate ganglion, located between the cog and the cochleariform process.

The stapes is then removed entering into the vestibule, exposing the saccule (**Fig. 4**A, B). The vestibule with the spherical recess in the saccular fossa are endoscopically detected, as the spherical recess is the end of the inferior vestibular nerve, representing an important landmark for the localization of the fundus of the IAC. The tegmen of the round window niche is removed carefully, exposing the membrane of the round window.

Using a Piezosurgery instrument (Mectron, Carasco/Genova, Italy), the promontory with lateral aspect of the otic capsule is removed at the cochlear level, identifying the basal, middle, and upper turn of the cochlea (**Fig. 4**C). After the exposition of the cochlear turns, the bony wall between the cochlea and the spherical recess is removed carefully, entering in the fundus of the IAC (**Fig. 4**D).

A dissection of the IAC is then progressively made, following the dura of the IAC from the fundus until the porus, exposing the AN (**Fig. 5**A). During this step, the bony tissue of the lateral skull is removed progressively between the IAC and the surrounding anatomic structures, exposing circumferentially the IAC. Respectively, the bony tissue between the IAC and the internal carotid artery anteriorly, the IAC and the mastoid portion of the facial nerve posteriorly, the IAC and the jugular bulb inferiorly, and the IAC and the tympanic segment of the facial nerve superiorly is removed, permitting a wide access to the IAC. The bony tissue of the otic capsule is removed

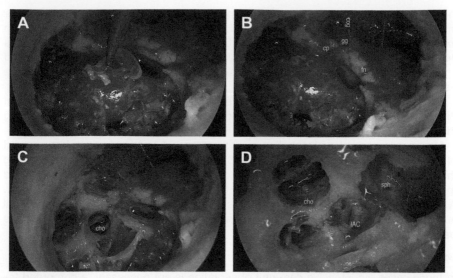

Fig. 4. Left ear; TTEA: (*A*) stapes is removed to expose the vestibule; (*B*) the vestibule now is opened and the tympanic portion of the facial nerve until the geniculate ganglion is under endoscopic view; (*C*) the promontory is progressively removed uncover the cochlear turns; (*D*) the fundus of the IAC is opened between the spherical recess and the cochlea. cho, cochlea; cp, cochleariform process; fn, facial nerve; gg, geniculate ganglion; IAC, internal auditory canal; sph, spherical recess.

from lateral to medial wall exposing the dura of the medial surface of the temporal bone, representing the deepest limit of the dissection.

After the IAC exposition, the dura of the IAC is opened and the neuroma into the canal is exposed (**Fig. 5**B). Before tumor removal, identification of the facial nerve

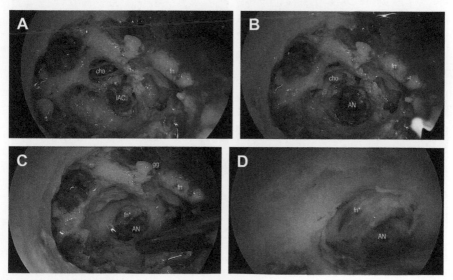

Fig. 5. Left ear; TTEA: (*A*) the IAC is skeletonized progressively; (*B*) the dura of the IAC is opened exposing the AN; (*C*) the facial nerve into the IAC is detected; (*D*) the AN is removed, preserving the facial nerve integrity. cho, cochlea; fn*, facial nerve into the IAC; gg, geniculate ganglion.

into the IAC is mandatory so as to avoid injury of the nerve (**Fig. 5C**). The stimulator of the facial nerve can help the surgeon during the detection of the nerve. After the exposition of the facial nerve into the IAC, the tumor is gently removed from the nerve and from the IAC using angled dissectors. The mass is gently dissected and removed in a piecemeal way, maintaining the integrity of facial nerve until the porus (**Fig. 5D**).

When the neuroma is showing a limited extension to the CPA, the bony opening of the porus can be enlarged using a diamond bur to gain access to the CPA, removing the last part of the tumor in the angle.

After tumor removal, an inspection is made of the IAC to confirm complete removal of the mass (**Fig. 6A–C**). Closure of the IAC is performed with abdominal fat, packing the promontorial defect and closing the communication between the inner ear and middle ear (**Fig. 6D**). A fibrin glue is used to fix the fat into the promontorial defect. A piece of muscle is used to close the Eustachian tube opening. The whole external auditory canal is filled with fat and a blind sac closure of the skin of the EAC is performed.

Postoperative Care

In these cases, an intensive care unit observation is not necessary, a computed tomography scan of the brain is performed 6 hours after the surgery (**Fig. 7**); the patient must be in supine position for 48 hours after surgery and if there are no complications, the patient is discharged after 4 days.

DISCUSSION

Retrosigmoid, middle cranial fossa, and transmastoid-translabyrinthine approaches are the most widely used in the traditional microscopic surgical removal of ANs.

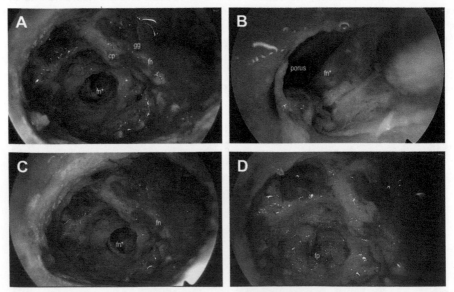

Fig. 6. Left ear; TTEA: (*A*) final cavity after AN removal; (*B*) a close view on the IAC until the porus after tumor removal; (*C*) the defect on the promontory area is detected; (*D*) a fat pad is used to close the promontorial defect. cp, cochleariform process; fn*, facial nerve into the IAC; fn, facial nerve; fp, fat pad; gg, geniculate ganglion.

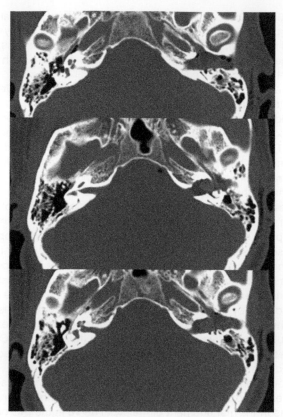

Fig. 7. Axial view CT scan after surgery on left ear showing the surgical route from the external to the internal auditory canal.

The retrosigmoid approach guarantees optimal control of the CPA, although its control of the IAC requires drilling of the posterior aspect of the petrous bone. In most cases, control of the fundus is very difficult to obtain.[10]

The middle cranial fossa approach is classically recommended for small ANs, because it guarantees limited access to the CPA, but for this approach a craniotomy with brain retraction is required, because the position of the IAC is in the superior aspect of the temporal bone; so that it cannot be used in large ANs extending widely outside the IAC.[10]

Both approaches, the retrosigmoid and middle cranial fossa, are chosen when hearing preservation is attempted, as occurs frequently for small ANs.[11]

Translabyrinthine approach guarantees a good exposure of both IAC and CPA, but results in a hearing loss and requires an extensive drilling of the petrous bone.[10]

All of these approaches necessitate wide external incisions and soft tissue dissection, craniotomy (retrosigmoid, middle cranial fossa), CPA exposure by cerebellar retraction (retrosigmoid), or temporal lobe retraction (middle cranial fossa) and extensive temporal bone drilling and tissue removal (translabyrinthine).

Complications associated with cerebellar dissection and retraction on the cerebellum with direct injury to the pial surface of the brain and venous infarcts and contusions observed in these traditional microscopic surgeries can be reduced leading to improved outcomes with the fully endoscopic technique, as a natural surgical corridor is used (EAC) to reach the IAC, from lateral to medial.

Because the fully endoscopic approach is through natural surgical corridor (EAC), the bony work is performed on the medial wall of the tympanic cavity and lateral skull base from lateral to medial, avoiding cerebellum and brain retractions. Therefore, this approach can be considered a minimally invasive procedure with low mobility if compared with other traditional surgery for AN removal.

For this, before starting with that kind of approach, several cadaver dissections were attempted to verify safety and reliability of the technique, and to understand surgical limits and landmarks.[9] It is anyway important that these procedures are performed by very experienced professionals, with years of training in endoscopic middle ear procedures. The skilled neurosurgeon must learn to work around the endoscope, often using techniques that have been borrowed from endonasal skull base surgery and are the natural evolution of middle ear endoscopic surgery.

Some key points of the procedure are herein pointed out. The first step of the procedure resembles middle ear approaches described in the past for cholesteatoma treatment, or for exploration and study of the middle ear.[4,6,12] Reaching the IAC from a surgical point of view, the main problem with the endoscopic technique is that in cases of some anterior inferior cerebellar artery branches or internal auditory artery bleeding, hemostasis would be very difficult to achieve in inexperienced hands; space is very limited compared with standard procedures. This issue is frequently emphasized by the scientific community discussing risks of exclusive endoscopic retrosigmoid procedures (by the "keyhole" technique). At present this is the main issue and criticism to the fully endoscopic approach, but it is possible to overcome the problem with a careful preoperative magnetic resonance (MR) study or CPA vascularization, and in cases in which unfavorable vascular anatomy is noticed, the approach should not be recommended.

Another consideration must be taken regarding the facial nerve dissection; it is well-known that the endoscopic technique is a "one-hand technique" requiring manual skills; for this reason the management of the facial nerve in the IAC could be difficult, especially when adhesion between the nerve and the tumor is found and careful surgical maneuvers are required to avoid damage to the nerve. For this purpose, knowledge of the surgical landmarks is mandatory for facial nerve preservation.

Indications for the technique are limited, as we have already mentioned before. Moreover, dealing with small ANs of the IAC, TTEA is an alternative to other options such as wait and scan policies or radiosurgery.

Actually, most small ANs do not grow,[13] and based on this fact a wait and scan policy is in most cases acceptable: this is particularly important if the hearing is not compromised. Anyway a late growing of the AN cannot be excluded in a life-span time, particularly in a patient with diagnosis made at early ages. In those cases, also hearing is very likely to deteriorate over time after decades. Moreover, in the "wait and scan" policy the patient must undergo to 6 months MR for the whole life. On the opposite, an older patient with a small AN could choose to avoid operation in favor of a wait and scan policy for the presence of comorbidities: we have to admit that the wait and scan policy is in most cases preferred because traditional AN surgeries are considered very delicate operations with possible risk of high morbilities and even a small risk of death. The fact that TTEA has a completely different route, and being an almost total extradural procedure with a morbidity comparable to a tympanoplasty, could probably change our attitude switching at least part of our choices from wait and scan procedures to surgery. The principle would be to operate until the AN is small by a minimally invasive approach, instead of waiting for the AN to grow so much that a minimally invasive approach could not be feasible anymore. All those considerations must find a confirmation by increasing the experiences and looking at the results over longer follow-ups, although in the present authors' feelings the TTEA seems very promising.

The debate about natural orifice transluminal surgery (NOTES) is nowadays in every sector of surgery[14] and the fully endoscopic approach for AN removal should be considered not only a minimally invasive procedure, but also a NOTES procedure.

The innovative endoscopic technique to the IAC and CPA completely change the traditional approaches and procedures to lateral skull base surgery, because it provides the adequate light and complete direct visualization of the masses that have to be removed and their relationship with the anatomic structures close or in contact with them.

As future prospective, a transcanal enlarge approach with the possibility to use the microscope through the EAC working with 2 hands using the same anatomic landmarks of the TTEA may be the natural evolution of this surgical technique, avoiding complications in the CPA, allowing sufficient working space to remove tumors involving the CPA with limited extension (Koos type 2 ANs).

SUMMARY

The exclusive fully endoscopic approach to the IAC removes ANs from the external to IAC without any external incisions. By this innovative approach, the complications observed in traditional microscopic surgeries can be reduced, with significantly shorter recovery time and hospitalization of the patients and possible improved outcomes on facial nerve. Indications for the fully endoscopic AN surgery are currently limited to pathology involving the anterior labyrinth and/or the IAC. These procedures should be performed by very experienced surgeons, with several years of training in endoscopic middle ear procedures.

REFERENCES

1. Magnan J, Chays A, Lepetre C, et al. Surgical perspectives of endoscopy of the cerebellopontine angle. Am J Otol 1994;15:366–70.
2. Shahinian HK, Ra Y. 527 fully endoscopic resections of vestibular schwannomas. Minim Invasive Neurosurg 2011;54:61–7.
3. Presutti L, Magnaguagno F, Pavesi G, et al. Combined endoscopic-microscopic approach for vestibular schwannoma removal: outcomes in a cohort of 81 patients. Acta Otorhinolaryngol Ital 2014;34:427–33.
4. Marchioni D, Alicandri-Ciufelli M, Molteni G, et al. Endoscopic tympanoplasty in patients with attic retraction pockets. Laryngoscope 2010;120:1847–55.
5. Marchioni D, Alicandri-Ciufelli M, Piccinini A, et al. Surgical anatomy of transcanal endoscopic approach to the tympanic facial nerve. Laryngoscope 2011;121: 1565–73.
6. Marchioni D, Villari D, Alicandri-Ciufelli M, et al. Endoscopic open technique in patients with middle ear cholesteatoma. Eur Arch Otorhinolaryngol 2011;268: 1557–63.
7. Marchioni D, Alicandri-Ciufelli M, Mattioli F, et al. From external to internal auditory canal: surgical anatomy by an exclusive endoscopic approach. Eur Arch Otorhinolaryngol 2013;270:1267–75.
8. Presutti L, Alicandri-Ciufelli M, Cigarini E, et al. Cochlear schwannoma removed through the external auditory canal by a transcanal exclusive endoscopic technique. Laryngoscope 2013;123:2862–7.
9. Marchioni D, Alicandri-Ciufelli M, Rubini A, et al. Endoscopic transcanal corridors to the lateral skull base: initial experiences. Laryngoscope 2015;125:S1–13.

10. Bennett M, Haynes DS. Surgical approaches and complications in the removal of vestibular schwannomas. Otolaryngol Clin North Am 2007;40:589–609.
11. Staecker H, Nadol JB Jr, Ojeman R, et al. Hearing preservation in acoustic neuroma surgery: middle fossa versus retrosigmoid approach. Am J Otol 2000;21: 399–404.
12. Marchioni D, Alicandri-Ciufelli M, Piccinini A, et al. Inferior retrotympanum revisited: an endoscopic anatomic study. Laryngoscope 2010;120:1880–6.
13. Patnaik U, Prasad SC, Tutar H, et al. The long-term outcomes of wait-and-scan and the role of radiotherapy in the management of vestibular schwannomas. Otol Neurotol 2015;36(4):638–46.
14. Berney CR. Natural orifice transluminal endoscopic surgery: where should we draw the line? Ann Surg 2011;254:1081–3.

Incorporating Endoscopic Ear Surgery into Your Clinical Practice

Elliott D. Kozin, MD[a,b], Ruwan Kiringoda, MD[a,b],
Daniel J. Lee, MD[a,b],*

KEYWORDS

- Endoscopic ear surgery • Neurotology • Cholesteatoma • Endoscope • EES
- Otology • Transcanal surgery

KEY POINTS

- Endoscopes allow for improved transcanal visualization of the tympanic cavity because the light source is located at the distal tip of the instrument, and angled optics offer a wide perspective of the operative field.
- For the right-handed surgeon, the authors recommend starting with left-sided transcanal endoscopic ear surgery (EES) cases because (1) the endoscope trajectory is ideal for visualizing disease in the posterosuperior mesotympanum and epitympanum, (2) the dissection instruments do not rest against the anterior canal wall, and (3) the camera hand can be rested against the patient's shoulder and bed.
- Until greater proficiency is achieved, the surgeon should always use the dominant hand for dissection.
- Room set-up and equipment position are crucial when beginning EES. To optimize ergonomics, a surgical chair with armrests should be used, and the video tower or boom-mounted video screen should be placed directly across from the surgeon and as close to eye level as possible.
- Essential equipment for EES includes a xenon, halogen, or light-emitting diode light source, rigid endoscopes (ideally, 14 cm in length and 3 mm in diameter), a high-definition (HD) 3-chip camera, and HD video monitor.

Disclosures: None.
Conflict of Interest: None.
[a] Department of Otolaryngology, Massachusetts Eye and Ear Infirmary, 243 Charles Street, Boston, MA 02114, USA; [b] Department of Otology and Laryngology, Harvard Medical School, Boston, MA, USA
* Corresponding author. Massachusetts Eye and Ear Infirmary, 243 Charles Street, Boston, MA 02114.
E-mail address: Daniel_Lee@meei.harvard.edu

Otolaryngol Clin N Am 49 (2016) 1237–1251
http://dx.doi.org/10.1016/j.otc.2016.05.005
0030-6665/16/$ – see front matter © 2016 Elsevier Inc. All rights reserved.

INTRODUCTION

Otologic surgery has progressed rapidly over the past century. Before the 1920s, ear surgery was completed either with loupes or without microscopic assistance. With the refinement of the binocular operating microscope in the 1950s, otologic surgery entered its modern era.[1,2] Until the 1990s, visualization of the tympanic cavity by surgeons was performed exclusively with operative microscopy (except by a handful of surgeons beginning in the 1960s), and approaches to the middle ear and mastoid were constrained by the surgeon's line of sight. Although modern microscopes provide excellent views of the surgical field, visualization of deeper recesses of the middle ear is limited. The optical properties of a microscope require an adequate amount of light to reach the surgical plane. Accordingly, microscope-based operative approaches frequently necessitate soft tissue retraction and/or bony drilling, such as mastoidectomy, to adequately visualize and access abnormality.

In contrast to microscopes, endoscopes allow for improved visualization because the light source is located at the distal tip of the instrument, and angled optics offer a wide perspective of the operative field. The use of endoscopy to visualize the middle ear was introduced in the late 1960s; however, poor image resolution in comparison to the operative microscope limited its application[3] (**Fig. 1**). With the introduction of 3-chip camera systems and high-definition (HD) video systems, endoscopes now provide ultrahigh resolution images of the middle ear never previously seen. Advocates of endoscopic ear surgery (EES) espouse its wide-field view, magnification, and the ability to look around corners. Furthermore, transcanal endoscopic ear surgery (TEES) approaches transform the external auditory canal into a minimally invasive surgical portal to access middle ear (and inner ear) disease (**Fig. 2**). It is important to emphasize that the endoscope is not meant to replace the microscope in all patients, but may serve a specialized purpose in select cases.

Initially, endoscopes were used in the ear predominately as an adjunct to microscopes for diagnostic purposes.[4,5] The improved image clarity, wide-angle view, and superior illumination of endoscopes afforded visualization of the middle ear cavity through transtympanic or transmastoid approaches with relative ease. Consequently, early studies on the application of endoscopes in middle ear surgery focused on the microanatomy of the middle ear. In the 1990s, as an extension of these anatomic studies, investigators examined the application of endoscopes as observational tools in cholesteatoma procedures to evaluate for residual or recurrent disease.[6–10] Recent studies from the past 10 years have demonstrated that the endoscope may be a reasonable alternative to the microscope to perform otologic surgery. Endoscopes revolutionized sinus surgery and may have a similar impact on otology for the following reasons:

1. *Visualization of middle ear anatomy is vastly improved with the endoscope.* The wide-angle and high-resolution image provided by the endoscope allows for improved visualization of the ear during surgery. This enhanced surgical view invites a more robust understanding of all middle ear structures and their spatial relationships.
2. *The endoscope expands the surgical reach of a transcanal approach to access complex middle disease.* EES transforms the external auditory canal into a minimally invasive portal for middle ear surgery (and inner ear surgery in selected cases).

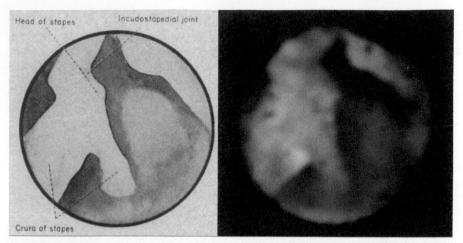

Fig. 1. Early endoscopic views of the middle ear, 1967. (*left panel*) Schematic showing endoscopic view of the stapes and incudostapedial joint. (*right panel*) Cadaveric view of stapes and incudostapedial joint using a custom-built rigid endoscope with roughly 2.5 mm diameter. (*From* Mer SB, Derbyshire AJ, Brushenko A, et al. Fiberoptic endotoscopes for examining the middle ear. Arch Otolaryngol 1967;85(4):387–93; with permission.)

Drawbacks of EES include a more challenging one-handed dissection and limited instrumentation. Modification of operative techniques and new instrumentation are needed to lower the barrier of adoption of EES.

In this review, the following are summarized: (1) surgical indications for EES, (2) proper surgical ergonomics, (3) necessary EES instrumentation, and (4) pearls and pitfalls associated with incorporating EES into your clinical practice.

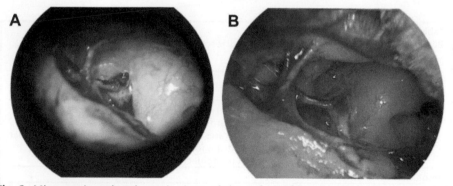

Fig. 2. Microscopic and endoscopic views of the right middle ear. This patient presented with right-sided conductive hearing loss and normal otoscopy. Intraoperative findings were consistent with spontaneous erosion of the incus. (*A*) Microscopic view of the right middle ear (patient is in supine position) taken at highest magnification with an HD 3-CCD video camera. (*B*) Endoscopic view of the same ear, demonstrating a wide-field view that has greater detail, depth, and clarity (0° endoscope, held in the *right* hand).

INDICATIONS FOR ENDOSCOPIC EAR SURGERY

The application of the endoscope to perform otologic surgery is currently debated, and indications are being refined (**Table 1**). Over the past decade, a handful of surgeons (mostly outside the United States) has used the endoscope as an instrument not only for observation but also as the sole instrument for visualization of the middle ear during operative dissection, similarly to the way paranasal sinus surgery is currently performed. Widespread acceptance of EES will rely on rigorous and prospective clinical outcomes, as well as standardization of surgical approaches, instrumentation, and nomenclature. At the Massachusetts Eye and Ear Infirmary (MEEI), a system to classify the use of endoscopy during otologic surgery (class 0–3; 0, no endoscope; 3, TEES) is being developed.[11] The classification system and subsequent modifications are examples of how to standardize operative descriptions and analyze clinical outcomes across large cohorts of patients and multiple institutions (**Table 2**).

Discrete indications for EES are growing rapidly, and the literature is rife with examples of emerging indications. Common applications of EES are described in **Box 1**. The authors strongly recommend attending an EES course to practice EES techniques in a temporal bone laboratory before trial in patients. The surgical views vary dramatically from microscope-based otologic cases, and transcanal techniques take practice to learn. Furthermore, most seasoned otologists may not have experience with endoscopic techniques developed for sinus surgery in the late 1990s. Practice with one-handed dissection in the controlled environment of a temporal bone laboratory is key. (If unable to attend a course, the authors encourage the use of a fresh cadaveric tissue, rather than fixed tissue, which better replicates pliable feel of the external auditory canal.)

The authors recommend a 3-step process to introduce EES into surgical practice:

1. Use the endoscope during chronic ear surgery *after* the microscopic-based dissection to
   a. Look for hidden disease

Table 1 Basic differences between endoscopic and microscopic ear surgery		
	Endoscope	**Microscope**
Number of hands Available for dissection	One-handed	Two-handed
Typical surgical approach	Transcanal (can be postauricular for combined cases as well as via the antrum following canal up mastoidectomy)	Transcanal with speculum ± endaural incision or postauricular
Resolution	High	High
Binocular vision	No	Yes
Field of view	Wide	Narrow
Ability to look around corners	Yes (0–70°)	No
Portal needed for visualization	Narrow	Wide

Table 2
Massachusetts Eye and Ear Infirmary Transcanal Endoscopic Ear Surgery classification system

	Description	TEES Vs. Non-TEES
Class 0	Operative microscope alone	Non-TEES
Class 1	Endoscope used for inspection/observation only; no dissection	
Class 2a	Mixed microscopic/endoscopic dissection; minority of dissection with endoscope	
Class 2b	Mixed microscopic/endoscopic dissection; majority of dissection with endoscope	
Class 2m	Endoscope-only case transitioned to microscopic case requiring mastoidectomy	
Class 3	Endoscope only (no operative microscope)	TEES

Adapted from Cohen MS, Landegger LD, Kozin ED, et al. Pediatric endoscopic ear surgery in clinical practice: lessons learned and early outcomes. Laryngoscope 2016;126(3):733; with permission.

Box 1
Indications for endoscopic ear surgery

External ear

- Cholesteatoma

- Exostosis repair

- Canalplasty

- Debridement and biopsy

Middle ear

- Myringotomy

- Myringoplasty

- Medial graft tympanoplasty

- Lateral graft tympanoplasty

- Tympanic membrane retraction

- Acquired cholesteatoma

- Congenital cholesteatoma

- Neoplasms of middle ear (eg, glomus tympanicum)

- Ossiculoplasty

Inner ear/skull base

- Intracochlear schwannoma

- Small symptomatic neoplasms of internal auditory canal (IAC) fundus or facial nerve

- Petrous apex cyst

- Perilymph fistula repair (congenital or traumatic)

Middle cranial fossa

- Superior canal dehiscence repair

Posterior fossa/cerebellopontine angle

- Identification of residual schwannoma in IAC fundus

- Localization and plugging of exteriorized air cells during IAC decompression to reduce cerebrospinal fluid leak risk

   b. Examine the retrotympanum, epitympanum, protympanum, and hypotympanum with a 30° endoscope
   c. Examine the antrum through the ear canal with a 30° endoscope
   d. Assess the ossicular chain and round window
2. Perform an "easy" transcanal procedure, including
   a. Endoscopic examination under anesthesia of the external canal and tympanic membrane before microscopic dissection to document abnormality
   b. Cerumen removal
   c. Tympanostomy tube placement
   d. Myringoplasty
3. Use the microscope to begin the tympanomeatal flap; then complete elevation with EES techniques
   a. Switch to a 0° endoscope before dissection of the annulus and then complete tympanotomy endoscopically

Do not expect to be able to perform a case from beginning to end using an endoscope while learning EES. Use the endoscope for limited aspects of cases. As experience is gained, do less with the microscope and more with the endoscope. Indeed, do not be concerned if you need to transition to a microscopic case, which is very common when starting EES (**Fig. 3**).

OPTIMIZED SURGICAL ERGONOMICS FOR ENDOSCOPIC EAR SURGERY

EES is a very challenging skill set to incorporate into an established otolaryngologic practice, and proper ergonomics are crucial to reduce the frustration and added operative time needed to develop proficiency with endoscopic cases. Proper body mechanics for EES is different from microscopic cases because surgeons will be watching a monitor versus using the binocular eyepieces of the microscope. Before the patient is brought into the room, surgeon, anesthesia, and ancillary operating staff must agree on the layout. In the case of need for conversion to a microscope-based case, the microscope should be readily accessible (**Table 3**).

Operating Room Setup

Fig. 4 demonstrates ideal positioning for left ear EES. The entire room layout is reversed for right-sided ear cases. To ensure minimal neck strain, the video tower (or boom-mounted video screen) should be directly across from the surgeon and placed as close to eye level as possible. The surgical scrub team should be placed across from the surgeon. The microscope should be placed in the corner of the room allowing for easy access.

The patient's head should be placed directly on the pad of the operating room table and one should NEVER place the head on a doughnut or headrest unless there is limited neck extension because this will limit the ability to rapidly use the microscope, if needed.

Hand Positioning and Placement of the Endoscope

Similar to standard otologic surgery, a chair that has armrests should be used. Both forearms/elbows should rest either on the table, patient shoulder, or armrest to maintain stability and minimize fatigue. The endoscope may be held in a similar fashion as endoscopic sinus surgery, which is partly along the shaft and camera head. The endoscope is proximally stabilized gently along the cartilaginous meatus. Note that any significant torque on the endoscope will bend the fiber-optic cable and reduce image quality. Some surgeons may stand during EES, similar to rhinologists during endo-scopic sinus surgery.

Left Versus Right Ears

Although EES reduces the visual limitations imposed by the anterior overhang of the external auditory canal, it does influence instrumentation of the middle ear (**Fig. 5**). Consequently, for the right-handed surgeon, the authors recommend starting with left-sided EES cases because dissection of routine and complex middle ear disease is much easier than the right ear. The 2 reasons for this are (1) the anterior canal over-hang does not limit access with dissection instruments and (2) the trajectory of the endoscope is biased toward the upper portion of the middle ear to allow for excellent visualization of the ossicles and facial nerve as well as access to most of middle ear disease. *The authors strongly recommend using the dominant hand for dissection in both left and right ear cases.* Left-handed surgeons are typically more ambidextrous, and one will find that switching hands may be easier when performing left ear surgery (using the left hand to hold the video camera and the right hand to dissect).

INSTRUMENTATION

Essential equipment for endoscopic middle ear surgery includes (1) a light source, (2) rigid endoscopes, 0° and 30° (45° is optional), (3) a HD 3-charge-coupled device (3-CCD) camera and video monitor.

Light Sources and Camera Systems

Light sources of varying brightness and temperature are readily available, including xenon, light-emitting diode (LED), and halogen. At MEEI, the authors typically use xenon light sources based on the quality of light and availability. Endoscope camera systems are available through a variety of venders. The main requirement for camera systems is a 3-CCD camera. Three-chip CCD cameras provide high resolution and clear video imaging quality by relying on individual CCDs for red, green, and blue light. (Single-chip cameras tend to "red out" and become saturated when used in a small area that contains bleeding.) Light source and camera systems are identical to that of modern sinus surgery, and thus, typically available in modern Otolaryngology oper-ating rooms.

Endoscopes

Currently, the Hopkins rod-lens system is a popular choice among Otolaryngologists and provides endoscopes of varying diameters, lengths, and angles of view. As the diameter expands, the image quality improves as more light is transmitted to the oper-ative field. However, the wider-diameter endoscopes decrease the working space available for additional instruments. The rigid endoscope diameters commonly used for ear surgery are 2.7 mm, 3 mm, and 4 mm. EES can be performed with 4-mm-diam-eter scopes if the external canal is large enough. Typical endoscope shaft lengths in EES are 11 cm, 14 cm, and 18 cm. At the MEEI, they prefer endoscopes that are 3 mm in diameter and 14 cm in length. Both 0° and 30° endoscopes are routinely used for most EES (**Fig. 6**).

Dissection Instruments

Currently, several manufacturers offer EES-specific dissectors. These EES-specific dissectors are not necessary to begin EES but are useful as the surgeon gains greater proficiency with this new technique. The basic otologic instrument tray is sufficient for

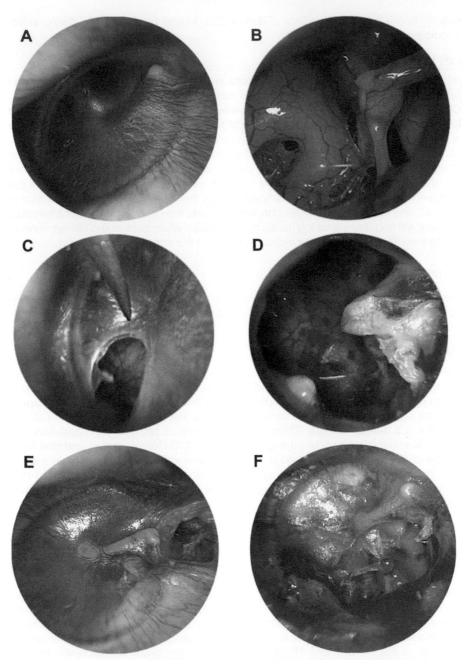

Fig. 3. Common external and middle ear findings in EES. (*A*) Left ear, 0° endoscope showing a normal tympanic membrane in a patient with conductive hearing loss. (*B*) Left ear, 0° endoscope showing completion of tympanotomy with view of ossicular chain, facial nerve, and cochlea following elevation of tympanomeatal flap from (*A*). This patient was found to have stapes fixation from otosclerosis (subtle white plaque seen anterior to stapes, in fissula ante fenestrum). (*C*) Left ear, 0° endoscope showing an inferior central perforation of the tympanic membrane, an ideal pediatric case for the beginning endoscopic ear surgeon.

Table 3
Operative equipment: differences between endoscopic and microscopic ear surgery

	Endoscope	Microscope
Source of visualization	Endoscope, 3-CCD camera, HD monitor	Microscope
Basic instrumentation	Standard otologic instrument set	Standard otologic instrument set
Additional instruments	Suction dissector, curved suction tips	None

most EES. Notably, the House-Crabtree dissector and House 20° incudostapedial joint knife, and a sharp stapes curette are specific instruments that are essential for EES dissection (**Figs. 7–9**).

Pearls and Pitfalls

There are several pearls and pitfalls that will be of great interest to the novice endoscopic ear surgeon:

- Proper trimming of ear hair is critical before the start of EES. The authors use a curved iris scissors under endoscopic guidance to ensure atraumatic removal. The endoscope may be replaced in the ear canal hundreds of times during a routine case. Hair will smudge the lens of the endoscope and require constant wiping.
- A useful way to way to hold the moist wipe and defog was originally described by Dr Ralph Metson, a pioneering sinus surgeon at MEEI. A microwipe saturated with saline and defog pad are each placed in a specimen container lid and secured near the ear of the patient (**Fig. 10**).
- Animal studies have indicated potential ototoxicity of defog solution, a combination of ethyl alcohol and surfactant.[12] The authors advise wiping the endoscope after application of defog with a saline-saturated microwipe or sponge to avoid introducing excessive defog solution in the middle ear.
- Flexible suction tubing will allow for freedom of movement that standard tubing may not afford (**Fig. 11**).
- The authors do not recommend the use of an endoscope holder.[13] If the patient moves during surgery, a fixed endoscope in the external or middle ear could damage the tympanic membrane or ossicular chain as the head moves laterally (and as both hands are holding either a suction or dissector, there would not be sufficient time to remove the endoscope quickly enough). In addition, most ear canals are unable to easily accommodate 3 instruments. For those surgeons with considerable skill with EES, a pneumatic endoscope holder may be considered in special circumstances only after discussion with the anesthesiologist regarding risk of patient movement during surgery. (Given that most otologic

(*D*) Left ear, 0° endoscope showing a child with a subtotal tympanic membrane perforation with cholesteatoma. This patient underwent a transcanal endoscopic lateral graft tympanoplasty with resection of disease. (*E*) Left ear, 0° endoscope showing attic cholesteatoma, an ideal indication for EES. (*F*) Left ear, 0° endoscope showing a dimeric tympanic membrane with complex retraction and perforation, incus erosion, and myringostapediopexy. This case is better suited for an experienced endoscopic ear surgeon or open approach. (*Courtesy of* [C] Michael Cohen, MD, Boston, MA.)

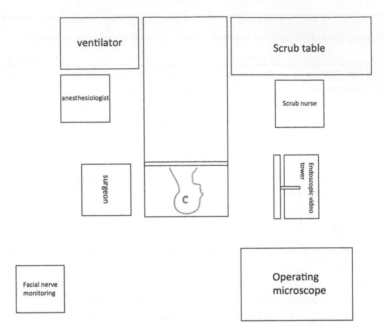

Fig. 4. EES room setup. The surgeon should be directly across from the endoscopic video tower (or boom-mounted video screen), which should be placed close to eye level to avoid neck strain. The scrub table can be placed at the foot of the bed to accommodate the video system. (*Adapted from* Kozin ED, Remenschneider AK, Shah PV, et al. Endoscopic transcanal removal of symptomatic external auditory canal exostoses. Am J Otolaryngol 2015;36:283–6; with permission.)

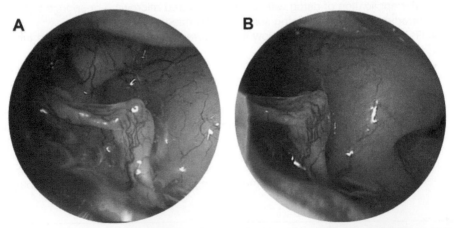

Fig. 5. Endoscopic view of the right middle ear changes with handedness of camera. This patient has a normal tympanic membrane on otoscopy and right-sided conductive hearing loss. Intraoperatively, spontaneous incus erosion was identified. (*A*) 0° endoscope held in the *right* hand provides a better view of the upper mesotympanum and ossicular chain and a small portion of the epitympanum (patient is supine). (*B*) 0° endoscope held in the *left* hand provides a better view of the lower mesotympanum with a better view of the round window niche.

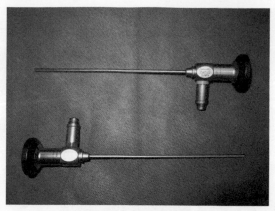

Fig. 6. Endoscopes designed for EES. 0° (*top*) and 30° (*bottom*), 3 mm diameter, 14-cm length rigid endoscopes. (Karl Storz, Tuttlingen, Germany.)

surgeries require facial nerve monitoring, patient paralysis is typically not feasible.)

- Similar to endoscopic sinus surgery, reverse Trendelenburg may result in decreased bleeding. In contrast to standard otologic surgery, position the patient in slight reverse Trendelenburg (~15°). Elevating the head will help to reduce

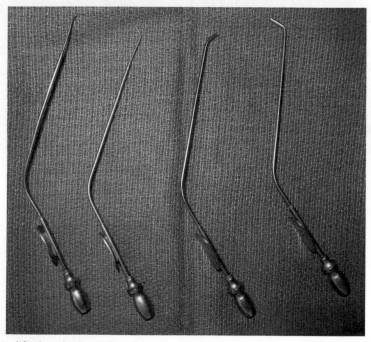

Fig. 7. Modified otologic suctions for EES. Existing suction instrumentation can be gently curved to reach areas that are visualized but not accessible with straight suctions. Bent 20-French and 5-French suction tips (up and down) are adequate for virtually all middle ear applications.

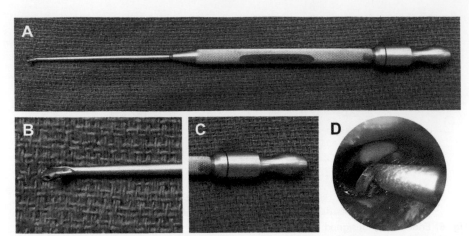

Fig. 8. Suction dissector. An essential tool for novice endoscopic ear surgeons to clear blood and secretions during one-handed dissection, if properly designed. (*A, B*) Modification of a traditional 2.5-mm-diameter round knife has microsuction in close proximity to the blade. (*C*) Swivel adapter to reduce kinking of tubing during dissection. (*D*) Properly designed suction dissector does not require the use of cottonoids to control hemostasis. (mytaMed, Malvern, PA.)

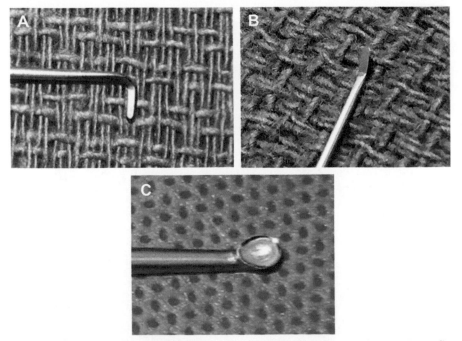

Fig. 9. EES instrumentation. (*A*) House-Crabtree dissector. This dissector has a 2.5-mm flattened tip and is angled at 90°. It is wonderfully designed to mobilize disease around corners and is ideally suited for EES. (*B*) 20° House Joint knife, which has slight angle and sharp (but rounded) tip for a variety of applications during endoscopic middle ear dissection. (*C*) Sharp stapes curette is the workhorse for bone removal during transcanal chronic ear surgery.

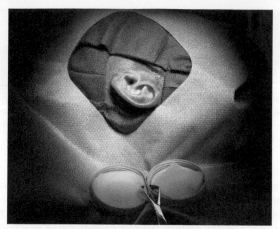

Fig. 10. Endoscope wipe and defog holder setup. A microwipe saturated with saline is better than a moist gauze sponge for streak-free wiping of the endoscope lens. Both the microwipe and the defog are placed in cup lids to reduce desiccation throughout surgery. Note: the microwipe is highly absorbent and will need repeated applications of saline.

bleeding during EES. Furthermore, similar to endoscopic sinus surgery, it is important to communicate with the anesthesiologist regarding blood pressure. Avoiding high blood pressure will also help to reduce bleeding.

- Injections with 1:10,000 lidocaine:epinephrine with a 27-gauge bent needle (**Fig. 12**) may also assist in hemostasis when raising a tympanomeatal flap. Cotton balls soaked in epinephrine may also be helpful to place in the canal along the edge of the flap. The authors suggest surgeons discuss with operating room staff, including anesthesiologists, before using nonstandard epinephrine mixtures. Continuous documentation of surgical counts of cotton balls during surgery is crucial to avoid leaving these items in the middle ear.
- Finally, several studies including research at MEEI in fresh human temporal bones have demonstrated the potential for high temperatures in the middle ear

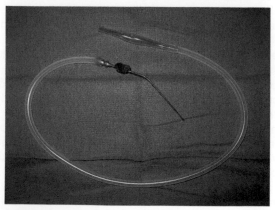

Fig. 11. Flexible suction tubing. A standard component to any otologic surgery, but given the additional technical challenges with EES, this is a must.

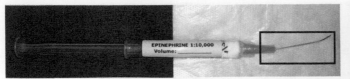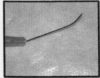

Fig. 12. Preparation of 27-gauge syringe needle for external auditory canal injection. Note double bend of needle tip that is essential to reach the lateral canal skin using the endoscope. The authors routinely use epinephrine (1:10,000–1:100,000) for vasoconstriction before raising the tympanomeatal flap.

associated with radiant energy from the endoscope.[14–17] For this reason, the authors recommend keeping the power of the light source no greater than 50% and a safe distance (>5 mm) away inner ear structures. In addition, frequently taking the endoscope out of the middle ear and coapplication of suction and irrigation are essential for cooling the middle ear space. Newer light sources, such as LED, may nominally reduce the heat transfer from the tip of the endoscope.

SUMMARY

Intraoperative use of the rigid endoscope is readily incorporated into the surgical practice with additional of minimal equipment and setup. Essential equipment for EES includes a light source, rigid endoscopes, a HD camera and video monitor, and angled suctions.

The MEEI "10 Commandments" of EES for the novice surgeon are as follows:

1. Participate in an EES course (or 2!) and practice in a temporal bone laboratory before beginning transcanal EES in your practice.
2. Essential EES surgery equipment to have available includes 0 and 30° endoscopes, 3-CCD HD camera, HD monitor, and standard otologic instrument set.
3. Discuss with the operating room team, including anesthesiologist and ancillary staff, the setup for EES before beginning any cases.
4. The light source should be no greater than 50% intensity to ensure patient safety.
5. For the right-handed surgeon, start with left-sided EES cases.
6. Trim ear canal hair before the start of EES cases to reduce smudging of endoscope lens.
7. Avoid using endoscope holders because these may cause an injury to middle ear anatomy in the event of unexpected patient movement.
8. Initial cases of EES include using the endoscope to look for hidden disease *after* using the microscope and then transitioning to "easy" procedures, including tympanoplasty tube placement and myringoplasty.
9. For angled endoscopes, *use two hands* to introduce the endoscope into the canal and middle ear: be aware of "blind spots" that may cause disruption of the ossicular chain. With practice, use one hand to hold the angled endoscope and the other hand to dissect.
10. Finally, keep practicing and expect setbacks: EES is technically challenging and may be frustrating in the first few cases, especially in regard to hemostasis. With greater proficiency, operating room times should be comparable or shorter than microscopic cases, especially if a postauricular incision is avoided.

REFERENCES

1. Uluc K, Kujoth GC, Baskaya MK. Operating microscopes: past, present, and future. Neurosurg Focus 2009;27(3):E4.
2. Mudry A. The history of the microscope for use in ear surgery. Am J Otol 2000;21: 877–86.
3. Mer S, Derbyshire J, Brushenko A, et al. Fiberoptic endotoscopes for examining the middle ear. Arch Otolaryngol 1967;85:61–7.
4. Nomura Y. Effective photography in otolaryngology-head and neck surgery: endoscopic photography of the middle ear. Otolaryngol Head Neck Surg 1982; 90:395–8.
5. Takahashi H, Honjo I, Fujita A, et al. Transtympanic endoscopic findings in patients with otitis media with effusion. Arch Otolaryngol Head Neck Surg 1990; 116:1186–9.
6. Yung M. The use of rigid endoscopes in cholesteatoma surgery. J Laryngol Otol 1994;108:307–9.
7. Thomassin J, Korchia D, Doris J. Endoscope-guided otosurgery in the prevention of residual cholesteatomas. Laryngoscope 1993;103:939–43.
8. Rosenberg S, Silverstein H, Hoffer M, et al. Use of endoscopes for chronic ear surgery in children. Arch Otolaryngol Head Neck Surg 1995;121:870–2.
9. Good G, Isaacson G. Otoendoscopy for improved pediatric cholesteatoma removal. Ann Otol Rhinol Laryngol 1999;108:893–6.
10. Haberkamp T, Tanyeri H. Surgical techniques to facilitate endoscopic second-look mastoidectomy. Laryngoscope 1999;109:1023–7.
11. Cohen MS, Landegger LD, Kozin ED, et al. Pediatric endoscopic ear surgery in clinical practice: lessons learned and early outcomes. Laryngoscope 2016; 126(3):732–8.
12. Nomura K, Oshima H, Yamauchi D, et al. Ototoxic effect of Ultrastop antifog solution applied to the guinea pig middle ear. Otolaryngol Head Neck Surg 2014; 151:840–4.
13. Kozin ED, Remenschneider AK, Shah P, et al. In response to: Letter to the editor. Am J Otol 2015;36:844–5.
14. Aksoy F, Dogan R, Ozturan O, et al. Thermal effects of cold light sources used in otologic surgery. Eur Arch Otorhinolaryngol 2015;272(10):2679–87.
15. Kozin E, Lehmann A, Carter M, et al. Thermal effects of endoscopy in a human temporal bone model: implications for endoscopic ear surgery. Laryngoscope 2014;124:E332–9.
16. MacKeith S, Frampton S, Pothier D. Thermal properties of operative endoscopes used in otorhinolaryngology. J Laryngol Otol 2008;122:711–4.
17. Tomazic P, Hammer G, Gerstenberger C, et al. Heat development at nasal endoscopes' tips: danger of tissue damage? A laboratory study. Laryngoscope 2012; 122:1670–3.

Endoscopic Techniques in Tympanoplasty

Jesus Franco Anzola, MD[a],*, João Flávio Nogueira, MD[b]

KEYWORDS

- Endoscopic ear surgery • Endoscopic tympanoplasty • Endoscopic myringoplasty
- Underlay • Overlay • Inlay • Interlay

KEY POINTS

- The endoscope allows improved view and reconstruction of tympanic membrane perforations.
- Endoscopic myringoplasty is feasible by a transcanal approach regardless of perforation size or anatomy of the ear canal.
- The endoscopic approach for tympanoplasty has not surpassed microscopic anatomic or functional outcomes, but it is undeniably less invasive and better tolerated by patients.
- Assessing the ventilation routes and preserving mastoid tissues may enhance functional outcomes for minimally invasive reconstruction of the middle ear.

 Video content accompanies this article at http://www.oto.theclinics.com.

INTRODUCTION

Tympanic membrane (TM) perforations are a common problem, most often as consequence of middle ear infection, traumatic rupture, or postoperative complication. Despite the autoregenerative capacity of the eardrum, chronic perforations may be subject to surgical repair.[1] The main goal of tympanoplasty (TP) is to restore anatomy and function and to eliminate disease; therefore, an uninterrupted TM, an air-containing mucosal-lined middle ear and a secure connection between the TM and the inner ear fluids are essential.[2,3]

The introduction of endoscopy to otologic surgery was underpinned by the ability to provide better access and view to otherwise hidden areas of the middle ear, such as the retrotympanum, anterior epitympanum, or middle ear folds, resulting in better appreciation of their relationships.[4–8] This improved visualization results from

[a] Otolaryngology & Skull Base Surgery, Centro Médico de Caracas. San Bernardino, Caracas 1010, Distrito Federal, Venezuela; [b] Sinus & Oto Centro, Hospital Geral de Fortaleza, Rua Dr. José Furtado 1480, Fortaleza 60822-300, Brazil
* Corresponding author.
E-mail address: jfrancoanzola@gmail.com

Otolaryngol Clin N Am 49 (2016) 1253–1264
http://dx.doi.org/10.1016/j.otc.2016.05.016
0030-6665/16/$ – see front matter © 2016 Elsevier Inc. All rights reserved.

closeness of the light source to the surgical field and wide angle optics, thereby transforming the external auditory canal into an excellent surgical portal.[9]

The endoscopic revolution has also lead to advances in anatomic and pathophysiologic concepts, which elucidate the role that middle ear folds play in blocking middle ear ventilation routes in patients with chronic otitis media. A more conservative approach preserving the mastoid tissues decreases morbidity and may improve postoperative middle ear ventilation, owing to their role in middle ear gas exchange. Systematic intraoperative visualization, analysis, and in some cases removal of these folds should be regarded as essential to restore middle ear physiology.[10–13] Endoscopes better illustrate these findings and aid in engaging this new philosophical perspective.

Endoscopic procedures, nevertheless, have several disadvantages. Given the diameter of the endoscope in relation to the ear canal, dissection may only be feasible with 1 hand and, thus, inefficient and challenging, chiefly when there is blood in the surgical field. Refinement of endoscopic skills and adopting precautionary hemostatic measures are paramount, a task more difficult to master by the surgeon with limited endoscopic training. Other caveats relate to heat dissipation and ototoxicity of antifog solutions.[14,15] Concern over thermal injury is warranted for elevated temperatures may occur up to 8 mm from the endoscope tip[15]; thus, smaller 3-mm endoscopes with submaximal light intensity (<60%), frequent removing–repositioning, irrigation of the surgical field, and suction are recommended.

Unlike the microscope that contemplates the surgical field from the outside, the endoscope itself is not immune to damage if unintentionally struck by a bone curette or a burr. Most instruments in use today were not customized for an endoscopic approach (EA), but rather migrated from traditional microscopic techniques; consequently, there will be a great demand for better and more refined tools in years to come.

Despite these potential drawbacks, the future of endoscopic ear surgery (EES) for minimally invasive functional reconstruction through a transcanal approach is enticing.

HAS THE ENDOSCOPE OUTPERFORMED THE MICROSCOPE?

In the narrow anatomy of the ear canal, surgery may be technically very demanding. To grant proper exposure, permeatal endaural incisions or postauricular approaches were used mainly for anterior and subtotal perforations and pediatric cases.[16] Without exception, all publications in the field agree that regardless of ear canal anatomy or age,[2,4,8,16–21] TP can be performed endoscopically through a transcanal approach. Increased postoperative pain, a numb or protruding pinna, and retroauricular scar or depression are frequently associated with more morbid approaches; therefore, a transcanal approach is preferred by patients because it grants improved comfort and aesthetics. As a result, endoscopic techniques for TP differ in 3 main aspects: (1) grafting material, (2) position of the graft in relation to the fibrous annulus and tympanic remnants, and (3) treatment of middle ear folds and ventilation routes.

Comparison of reported surgical outcomes between the endoscope and microscope may be explained not only by technique variants or differences in patients underlying pathology, age, or risk factors, but by the sole definition of success. Normal middle ear function after TP clearly requires more than an intact graft. An imperforate lateralized graft in the middle of the ear canal or a "Kevlar-armored" cartilage graft with poor audiological outcomes are equally undesirable. Therefore, a stricter definition of success, including anatomic and functional criteria as well as prevention of complications, has been promoted, even when confronted with more modest results (**Box 1**).[22]

Box 1
Recommended criteria for success in tympanoplasty

1. Anatomic success
   a. Intact graft without perforation or lateralization.

2. Functional success
   a. Improvement in hearing by assessing the ABG of less than 20 dB (0.5–3 kHz) or conservation of hearing (if normal preoperative audiometry).
   b. Aerated middle ear space (TM in normal anatomic position).

3. Prevent complications
   a. Ossicular disruption or acoustic trauma.
   b. Taste disturbance (chorda tympani injury).
   c. Neurovascular injury.

Abbreviations: ABG, air–bone gap; TM, tympanic membrane.

Complications have yet to be reported on endoscopic TP; EES is very anatomic and, as such, should bestow little trauma to the middle ear. The overzealous surgeon may misuse this tremendous advantage by inordinate manipulation around the ossicular chain when treating the middle ear folds and ventilation routes. Rarely, taste disturbance may result from traction or section of the chorda tympani.[23–25]

Given the logical learning curve for EET, one would expect lengthier surgical times and hospital stays, but no significant change has been reported; better yet, it may be even faster.[17] This suggests a steeper learning curve for otologic surgeons acquainted with endoscopic sinus surgery.[18]

Several notable studies have directly compared anatomic and functional success for in TP by an EA or microscopic approach (MA). Very similar graft survival (MA 83%–86% vs EA 83.3%–90%) and functional success rates (MA 85%–90% vs EA 90%) have been reported in adults, using an underlay technique (fascia or perichondrium).[19–21]

Dundar and colleagues[2] compared 32 EA with 29 MA for type I TP in children using a cartilage–perichondrial graft by the underlay technique, with compatible graft success (MA 93.1% vs EA 87.5%) and air–bone gap gain (MA 13 dB vs EA 12.2 dB). Cohen and colleagues[21] compared outcomes after 13 EA versus 19 MA type 1 myringoplasties in a pediatric cohort. No differences in graft closure (MA 84.6% vs 78.9% EA; $P>.99$), mean PTA threshold improvement (MA 27.8 dB vs EA 21.33 dB) or surgical time where shown. In a retrospective study, Nader and colleagues[17] compared 23 MA versus 22 EA, using an underlay technique in children (5–16 years old), with anatomic success at the 1-year follow-up of 82.6% for MA versus 90.9% for EA ($P>.05$). No difference in preoperative or postoperative air–bone gap values, bone threshold impairment, or postoperative complications was observed between the groups.

TP in children is often regarded as being less successful because of their higher propensity to infection, impaired Eustachian tube function, and adenoidal tissue hypertrophy.[26–28] In the endoscopic era, previous adenotonsillectomy, active infection, auditory tube dysfunction, perforation size, and age have not been reported as negative prognostic factors for pediatric TP.[29]

Surgical treatment of middle ear folds for clearing middle ear ventilation routes up to the mastoid cell system is the backbone of EES philosophy. Postoperative improvements in gas exchange and overall middle ear physiology converges on this premise. The anatomy of the epitympanic diaphragm, spectrum of pathologic variants, and their dynamic sequelae are somewhat perplexing. Marchionni and colleagues[8,10] have shed light on the subject describing 3 different types of TP in patients with selective epitympanic dysventilation syndromes with encouraging results. Several questions have yet to be answered: (1) Can surgery warrant isthmus permeability in the long term? (2) Inlay, interlay, and overlay techniques cannot properly address this problem; how does that affect outcomes and patient selection? (3) Underlay grafting may decrease not only middle ear space but narrow the anterior isthmus (as frequently observed in revision cases), does this justify over–under grafting as instead?

ENDOSCOPIC TYMPANOPLASTY AND GRAFTING SELECTION

The TM repairs mainly by epithelial migration, grafting materials act as scaffolds to guide the cell migration from the edges of the perforation, facilitating closure by providing a patch on which the neomembrane grows.[30,31] Because TM must heal by secondary intention, the size and location of the perforation may influence the results.[32,33]

Anatomic and physiologic factors might contribute toward a less favorable prognosis for graft survival in anterior quadrant and marginal perforations as a result of vascular supply, metabolic activity, and inadequate graft support.[34] Fluorescein angiography has shown a more vigorous vascular supply for the posterior TM[35] and a greater metabolic demand at the anterior annulus could explain the greater risk for necrosis and delayed healing. Specific technical difficulties in repairing anterior perforations as a bulging canal wall or the lack of a structure to support the graft anteriorly may also lead to poorer outcomes. Complete visualization of the TMP and surrounding annular rim, as well as correct graft placement are requirements well-suited for the EA. Most of the time, transcanal endoscopy avoids canalplasty, even for anterior or total perforations.[36]

Recently, there have been reports of an 87.5% to 95.5% TM closure and 91% functional success (6.4–8.5 dB air–bone gap gain) for anterior perforations grafted with cartilage by an expeditious totally endoscopic transcanal inlay butterfly or (**Fig. 1**) pushthrough technique.[37,38]

Temporalis Muscle Fascia

Temporalis muscle fascia (TMF) remains the gold standard in the clinical practice and the main reference against which other grafting materials are compared. The TMF microstructure is pliable and abundant; however, its shrinkage can be unpredictable because the gaps between its elastic fibers are filled with connective tissue that shrinks and thickens more than elastic fibers do.[36] Graft success rates of EA range between 82% and 93% and are consonant with the 80% of 10-year follow-ups of both underlay and overlay microscopic techniques.[39] A soft TMF is difficult to unfold and arrange inside the ear canal; a useful surgical pearl is to fix the graft's edge against the ear canal with the endoscope tip while unfolding with the other hand.

Cartilage and Perichondrium

As opposed to other grafts, cartilage provides a more robust scaffold, and is well-tolerated by the middle ear because it induces little tissue inflammation, resists infection during the recovery process, and can be viable even after delayed epithelization owing to its bradytrophic properties and nourishment by diffusion.[30,32] It first became the preferred grafting material for advanced middle ear pathologies when an increased risk of Eustachian tube dysfunction was expected,[40] paving the way for its widespread use in large perforation and primary low-risk cases; hearing results have shown to be comparable to tragal perichondrium and TMF.[29,41] Dornhoffer's[42] 1000 TP series using cartilage grafts proved to have a very low recurrence rate of 4.2%, even though

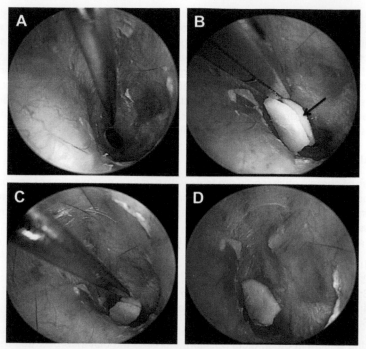

Fig. 1. Endoscopic inlay technique with a cartilage butterfly graft. (*A*) Edges of a small anterior perforation are refreshed. (*B*) Cartilage is shaped 2 mm larger than the perforation and a 1-mm groove is carved on its perimeter (*black arrow*). (*C, D*) Graft is fixed, anterior segment first, in analogy to a ventilation tube.

47% were revision cases. Whenever risk factors for graft failure are identified (subtotal or anterior perforations,[33,43] significant inflammatory changes in middle ear mucosa or contralateral ear pathology[24]), an alternative durable graft material such as cartilage must be considered.[40]

Cartilage is also versatile, because it can be used with or without perichondrium as a shield, island (single or bipedicled), palisade, or plug. For endoscopic purposes, it is much easier to allocate with 1 hand and can also be easily harvested from the tragus. High graft take rates have been published for EA in both adults (87.5%–96%) and children (88%–100%).[29,37,38,44–49]

The characteristics of cartilage are worse than more pliable tissues because of its thickness, rigidity,[50,51] and potential restriction of middle ear space. Experiments using variable cartilage thickness have shown that split thickness grafts of 0.5 mm or less have acceptable acoustic transfer with good mechanical stability.[1,52] In the clinical setting, however, there has been some controversy as to whether slicing the cartilage graft is necessary to attain optimal hearing results.[31,50,53] Another limitation of cartilage grafting is losing the apparent translucency of the membrane; therefore, otoscopy is unreliable for postoperative documentation of recurrent cholesteatoma or middle ear effusion.

Fat

Autologous fat has received attention as a safe and effective material for inlay grafting in small TMP with success rates between 76% and 92%, similar to those of TMF and paper patch.[32] Additionally, fat grafts secrete angiogenic growth factors that promote neovascularization and tissue repair, thus increasing the scanty blood supply around the TMP.[30] Earlobe and subcutaneous retroauricular fat are quickly obtained with low morbidity, but fat supply is poor, and so generous sources like abdominal fat have been promoted.[54,55] In medium or large pars tensa perforations of more than 30%, most authors agree that success rates decrease with fat grafting.[56,57] There are no reports in the literature on outcomes after endoscopic inlay fat myringoplasty.

Despite the large variety of scaffolds and surgical techniques available there is still no consensus on the optimal alternative for the TM repair. Thus, new therapeutic approaches are needed to overcome these drawbacks.[32]

SURGICAL TECHNIQUE

Each case of chronic otitis media presents with a unique combination of anatomic deficits, impaired function, unrelenting infection, and expectations for improvement. The art of surgery is to choose appropriately among different techniques to provide the best possible result.

There are 5 steps to every endoscopic TP:

Step 1: Optimizing hemostasis.
Step 2: Graft harvest.
Step 3: Preparing the TM and middle ear approach.
Step 4: Ossicular chain and ventilation routes assessment.
Step 5: Grafting.

Place the patient in otosurgical position, increase the distance between the shoulder and pinna to improve ergonomics. A 0° or 30°, 3 × 110 to 140-mm rigid endoscope is used throughout most of the surgery, whereas a 45° endoscope is advised to assess the retrotympanum, protympanum, and ventilation routes.

Step 1: Optimizing Hemostasis

- Gently infiltrate the ear canal and graft donor site with a 1:100,000 epinephrine + 2% lidocaine solution.
- Cottonoids soaked in 1:2000 epinephrine are left adjacent to the TM for 10 minutes, while graft is being harvested.
- Total intravenous anesthesia is preferred with a targeted mean blood pressure of 60 mm Hg and heart rate of 60 bpm.

Step 2: Graft Harvest

- Tragal perichondrium and cartilage
  - Incise the posterior edge of the tragus leaving a 2-mm rim of cartilage for cosmesis.
  - Thin undersurface tragal perichondrium is well-suited for overlay or underlay techniques, whereas the sturdier anterior perichondrium is used with cartilage as a tailored composite graft for scutum reconstruction.
  - Cartilage is cut to fit as a shield, island, palisade, or butterfly inlay graft.
- TMF is harvested through a retroauricular incision and pressed, not dehydrated, for ease of handling.
- Subcutaneous retroauricular tissue, earlobe or umbilical region fat, should double in size that of the TMP.

Step 3: Preparing the Tympanic Membrane and Approach to the Middle Ear

- Refresh TMP edges. Include the mucoepithelial junction.
- Abrade the tympanic undersurface for underlay techniques.

- Endocanal or transcanal approach the middle ear:
  - Endocanal: (without tympanomeatal flap).
    - A simple underlay "pushthrough" technique with a TMF, perichondrium, or an oval-shaped cartilage island graft is favored for small TMP. The graft is placed against TMP edges with fibrin glue or by previous filling the middle ear with absorbable gelatin sponges. Inlay fat or butterfly cartilage (2-mm larger than TMP) are placed analogous to a ventilation tube (Video 1)
  - Transcanal technique (**Figs. 2** and **3**):
    - Elevate a broad front tympanomeatal flap. Extend the superior limb past the 12 o'clock position to avoid inadvertent pars flaccida tears and ease to dissect from the malleolar lateral process.
    - Initial bleeding, limited support for the optics, and ample tilting to view the more tenacious fibers of the superior canal skin make this step technically challenging.

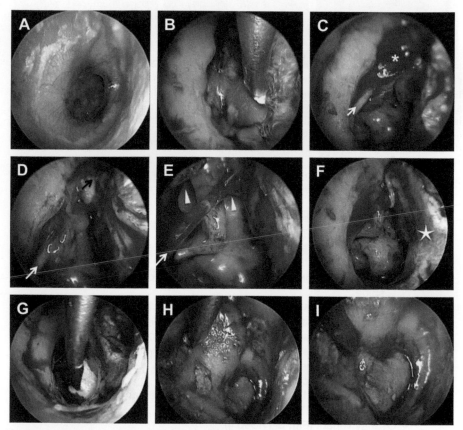

Fig. 2. Endoscopic underlay technique. (*A*) Central perforation, mucoepithelial junction is resected and a broad tympanomeatal flap is elevated up to the annular ligament (*B*). Chorda tympani (*white arrow*) is engulfed by thick inflammatory tissue (*asterisk*) closing ventilation routes (*C*). Gentle dissection exposes Prussak's space (*black arrow; D*), and the isthmus (*yellow arrowheads; E*). A perichondrium graft is placed under the tympanic remnant (*white star; F*), the middle ear packed with absorbable gelatin sponges (*G*). Juxta-position of the graft and tympanic remnant are verified (*H, I*).

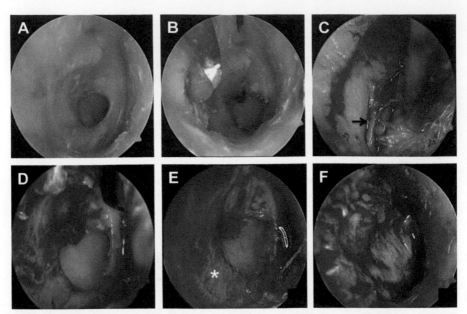

Fig. 3. Overlay endoscopic myringoplasty. (*A*) Central perforation is inspected and edges refreshed. (*B*) A short flap is elevated in proximity to the annular ligament (*black arrow; C*), and the epithelial layer of the tympanic membrane is carefully separated (*D*) from its fibrous layer up to the anterior annulus (*D*). No epithelium remains over the tympanic remnant (*asterisk*) (*E*). A perichondrial graft is placed over the drum (*F*) and the epithelial layer draped over it (interlay technique).

- Slide a small, epinephrine-soaked cottonoid or sponge against the canal wall, under the flap with a 3-F suction, to maintain flap integrity and hemostasis.
- Identify the posterior annulus.
  - Underlay variant (**Fig. 2**) (Videos 2 and 3):
    - Carefully lift the annulus from the sulcus. Identify and leave the chorda tympani unharmed.
    - Detach the posterior malleolar ligament from the posterior tympanic spine.
    - Expose Prussak's space and separate the pars flaccida from Rivinus' notch by gentle anterior traction with an alligator forceps.
    - Remove the cartilage cap of the lateral process with a sickle knife and proceed with subperiostial dissection between the TM and malleolar handle up to the umbo. If further exposure is needed, divide the final ligament with microscissors.
    - Retract the TM forward; inspect the middle ear spaces and tympanic diaphragm.
  - Overlay variant (**Fig. 3**) (Video 4):
  - Without lifting the annulus, dissect the epithelial layer from the fibrous drum until the anterior annulus is reached. Discard the epithelial layer (overlay) or save to partially cover the graft (interlay).

Step 4: Ossicular Chain and Ventilation Routes Assessment

- The ossicular chain is inspected and reconstruction is executed when necessary.

- Corroborate permeability of the anterior and posterior isthmus. Inspect the tensor fold from underneath placing the endoscope anterior to malleus' handle or from above after removal of the incus and head of malleus (**Fig. 3**C-E).
- If the isthmus is patent and there is no evidence of epitympanic retraction pockets or cholesteatoma the tensor fold does not need to be opened.

Step 5: Grafting

- Overlay: the graft is allocated over the fibrous tympanic remnant, and covered with saline soaked absorbable gelatin sponges (**Fig. 3**F).
- Underlay (**Fig. 2**):
  - ○ Fill the middle ear with absorbable gelatin sponges. A large protympanum may require more to support the graft, but avoid overpacking.
  - ○ Place the graft under the malleus and drape the native drum remnant over it. Confirm that all the epithelium is unfurled and there are no gaps.
    - ■ Over–under variant (Video 5):
      - To preserve the middle ear cleft space, especially if the malleus is retracted towards the promontory, the graft (cartilage or composite) may be arranged under the tympanic remnant but over the malleus handle.
      - Lay small pieces of absorbable gelatin sponges over the reconstructed TM.

SUMMARY

The endoscope has transformed the way we observe, understand, and treat chronic ear disease. Improved view, exclusive transcanal techniques, assessment of ventilation routes and mastoid tissue preservation have led to decreased morbidity and functional enhancement of minimally invasive reconstruction of the middle ear. EES' philosophical identity is evolving; new research, long-term results, and widespread acknowledgement of its postulates will undoubtedly define its role in otology.

SUPPLEMENTARY DATA

Supplementary data related to this article can be found online at http://dx.doi.org/10.1016/j.otc.2016.05.016.

REFERENCES

1. Volandri G, Di Puccio F, Forte P, et al. Biomechanics of the tympanic membrane. J Biomech 2011;44:1219–36.
2. Dundar R, Kulduk E, Soy FK, et al. Endoscopic versus microscopic approach to type 1 tympanoplasty in children. Int J Pediatr Otorhinolaryngol 2014;78:1084–9.
3. Fayad J, Sheehy J. Tympanoplasty-Outer outer surface grafting technique. Otologic Surgery 2010;9:119–27.
4. Presutti L, Marchioni D, Mattioli F, et al. Endoscopic management of acquired cholesteatoma: our experience. J Otolaryngol Head Neck Surg 2008;37:481–7.
5. Marchioni D, Mattioli F, Alicandri-Ciufelli M, et al. Endoscopic approach to tensor fold in patients with attic cholesteatoma. Acta Otolaryngol 2009;129:946–54.
6. Marchioni D, Mattioli F, Alicandri-Ciufelli M, et al. Transcanal endoscopic approach to the sinus tympani: a clinical report. Otol Neurotol 2009;30:758–65.
7. Tarabichi M. Endoscopic management of limited attic cholesteatoma. Laryngoscope 2004;114(7):1157–62.

8. Marchioni D, Mattioli F, Alicandri-Ciufelli M, et al. Endoscopic evaluation of middle ear ventilation route blockage. Am J Otolaryngol 2010;31(6):453–66.

9. Kozin ED, Gulati S, Kaplan AB, et al. Systematic review of outcomes following observational and operative endoscopic middle ear surgery. Laryngoscope 2015;125:1205–14.

10. Marchioni D, Alicandri-Ciufelli M, Molteni G, et al. Endoscopic tympanoplasty in patients with attic retraction pockets. Laryngoscope 2010;120:1847–55.

11. Doyle WJ. The mastoid as a functional rate-limiter of middle ear pressure change. Int J Pediatr Otorhinolaryngol 2007;71:393–402.

12. Sade J, Ar A. Middle ear and auditory tube: middle ear clearance, gas exchange, and pressure regulation. Otolaryngol Head Neck Surg 1997;116:499–524.

13. Takahashi H, Sato H, Nakamura H, et al. Correlation between middle-ear pressure-regulation functions and outcome of type-I tympanoplasty. Auris Nasus Larynx 2007;34:173–6.

14. Kozin ED, Lehmann A, Carter M, et al. Thermal effects of endoscopy in a human temporal bone model: implications for endoscopic ear surgery. Laryngoscope 2014;124(8):E332–9.

15. Nomura K, Oshima H, Yamauchi D, et al. Ototoxic effect of ultrastop antifog solution applied to the guinea pig middle ear. Otolaryngol Head Neck Surg 2014; 151(5):840–4.

16. Kessler A, Potsic WP, Marsh RR. Type I tympanoplasty in children. Arch Otolaryngol Head Neck Surg 1994;120:487–90.

17. Nader N, Berlucchi M, Redaelli de Zinis LO. Tympanic membrane perforation in children: endoscopic type I tympanoplasty, a newly technique, is it worthwhile? Int J Pediatr Otorhinolaryngol 2015;79(11):1860–4.

18. Raj A, Mejer R. Endoscopic transcanal myringoplasty: a study. Indian J Otolaryngol Head Neck Surg 2001;53(1):47–9.

19. Hagurop AS, Mudhol RS, Godhi RA. A comparative study of endoscope assisted myringoplasty and microscope assisted myringoplasty. Indian J Otolaryngol Head Neck Surg 2008;99(2):298–302.

20. Lade H, Choudhary SR, Vashishth A. Endoscopic vs microscopic myringoplasty: a different perspective. Eur Arch Otorhinolaryngol 2014;271:1897–902.

21. Cohen MS, Landegger LD, Kozin ED, et al. Pediatric endoscopic ear surgery in clinical practice: lessons learned and early outcomes. Laryngoscope 2016; 126(3):732–8.

22. Committee on Hearing and Equilibrium guidelines for the evaluation of results of treatment of conductive hearing loss. American Academy of Otolaryngology–Head and Neck Surgery Foundation, Inc. Otolaryngol Head Neck Surg 1995; 113:186–7.

23. Karatayli-Ozgursoy S, Ozgursoy OB, Muz E, et al. Evaluation of taste after underlay technique myringoplasty using whole mouth gustatory test: smokers versus non smokers. Eur Arch Otorhinolaryngol 2009;266:1025–30.

24. Mueller CA, Khatib S, Naka A, et al. Clinical assessment of gustatory function before and after middle ear surgery: a prospective study with a two year follow-up period. Ann Otol Rhinol Laryngol 2008;117:769–77.

25. Ciofalo A, Zambetti G, Romero M, et al. Taste and olfaction in middle ear surgery. Ann Otol Rhinol Laryngol 2015;124(4):312–3.

26. Yung M, Neumann C, Vowler SL. A longitudinal study on pediatric myringoplasty. Otol Neurotol 2007;28(3):353–5.

27. Caylan R, Titiz A, Falcioni M, et al. Myringoplasty in children: factors influencing surgical outcome. Otolaryngol Head Neck Surg 1998;118(5):709–13.

28. Vrabec JF, Deskin RW, Grady JJ. Meta-analysis of pediatric tympanoplasty. Arch Otolaryngol Head Neck Surg 1999;125(5):530–4.
29. Awad OG, Hamid KA. Endoscopic type 1 tympanoplasty in pediatric patients using tragal cartilage. JAMA Otolaryngol Head Neck Surg 2015;141(6):532–8.
30. Teh BM, Marano RJ, Shen Y, et al. Tissue engineering of the tympanic membrane. Tissue Eng Part B Rev 2013;19:116–32.
31. Vashishth A, Mathur M, Verma D. Cartilage palisades in type 3 tympanoplasty: functional and hearing results. Indian J Otolaryngol Head Neck Surg 2014; 66(3):309–13.
32. Villar-Fernández M, Lopez-Escamez JA. Outlook for tissue engineering of the tympanic membrane. Audiol Res 2015;5(1):117.
33. Lee P, Kelly G, Mills RP. Myringoplasty: does the size of the perforation matter? Clin Otolaryngol Allied Sci 2002;27(5):331–4.
34. Gerdsdroff M, Garin P, Decat M, et al. Myringoplasty: long–term results in adults and children. Am J Otol 1995;16(4):532–5.
35. Applebaum LL, Deutsch FC. An endoscopic method of tympanic membrane fluorescein angiography. Ann Otol Rhinol Laryngol 1986;95:439–43.
36. Ayache S. Cartilaginous myringoplasty: the endoscopic transcanal procedure. Eur Arch Otorhinolaryngol 2013;270:853–60.
37. Celic H, Samim E, Oztuna D. Endoscopic "push-trough" technique cartilage myringoplasty in anterior tympanic membrane perforations. Clin Exp Otorhinolaryngol 2015;8(3):224–9.
38. Eren SB, Tugrul S, Ozucer B, et al. Endoscopic transcanal inlay myringoplasty: alternative approach for anterior perforations. Otolaryngol Head Neck Surg 2015;153(5):891–3.
39. Nardone M, Sommerville R, Bowman J, et al. Myringoplasty in simple chronic otitis media: critical analysis of long-term results in a 1,000-adult patient series. Otol Neurotol 2012;33:48–53.
40. Hartzell LD, Dornhoffer JL. Timing of tympanoplasty in children with chronic otitis media with effusion. Curr Opin Otolaryngol Head Neck Surg 2010;18(6):550–3.
41. Mohamad SH, Khan I, Hussain SSM. Is cartilage tympanoplasty more effective than fascia tympanoplasty? Otol Neurotol 2012;33:699–705.
42. Dornhoffer JL. Cartilage tympanoplasty: indications, techniques and outcomes in a 1000 patient series. Laryngoscope 2003;113:1844–56.
43. Boronat-Echeverría NE, Reyes-García E, Sevilla-Delgado Y, et al. Prognostic factors of successful tympanoplasty in pediatric patients: a cohort study. BMC Pediatr 2012;12:67.
44. Yadav SP, Aggarwal N, Julaha M, et al. Endoscope assisted myringoplasty. Singapore Med J 2009;50(5):510.
45. Mohindra S, Panda NK. Ear surgery without microscope; is it possible. Indian J Otolaryngol Head Neck Surg 2010;62(2):138–41.
46. Yung M, Vivekanandan S, Smith P. Randomized study comparing fascia and cartilage grafts in myringoplasty. Ann Otol Rhinol Laryngol 2011;40:295–9.
47. Cabra J, Moñux A. Efficacy of cartilage palisade tympanoplasty: randomized controlled trial. Otol Neurotol 2010;31:589–95.
48. Migirov L, Wolf M. Transcanal microscope-assisted endoscopic myringoplasty in children. BMC Pediatr 2015;15:32.
49. Venegas M, Morante JC. Transcanal endoscopic tympanoplasty with tragal perichondrium graft by the under-over. Otolaryngol Head Neck Surg 2013;149(Suppl 2):P238.

50. Mokbel KM, Thabet el SM. Repair of subtotal tympanic membrane perforation by ultrathin cartilage shield: evaluation of take rate and hearing result. Eur Arch Otorhinolaryngol 2013;270:33–6.
51. Zang Z, Huang QH, Zheng YQ, et al. Three autologous substitutes for myringoplasty: a comparative study. Otol Neurotol 2011;32:1234–8.
52. Aernouts J, Soons JA, Dirckx JJ, et al. Quantification of tympanic membrane elasticity parameters from in situ point indentation measurements: validation and preliminary study. Hear Res 2010;263:177–82.
53. Gerber MJ, Mason JC, Lambert PR. Hearing results after primary cartilage tympanoplasty. Laryngoscope 2000;110(12):1994–9.
54. Kwong KM, Smith MM, Coticchia JM. Fat graft myringoplasty using umbilical fat. Int J Pediatr Otorhinolaryngol 2012;76:1098–101.
55. Acar M, Yazıcı D, San T, et al. Fat-plug myringoplasty of ear lobule vs abdominal donor sites. Eur Arch Otorhinolaryngol 2015;272(4):861–6.
56. Gun T, Sozen T, Boztepe OF, et al. Influence of size and site of perforation on fat graft myringoplasty. Auris Nasus Larynx 2014;41(6):507–12.
57. Konstantinidis I, Malliari H, Tsakiropoulou E, et al. Fat myringoplasty outcome analysis with otoendoscopy: who is the suitable patient? Otol Neurotol 2013; 34(1):95–9.

Endoscopic Management of Attic Cholesteatoma
Long-Term Results

Matteo Alicandri-Ciufelli, MD, FEBORL-HNS[a,b,]*,
Daniele Marchioni, MD[c], Seiji Kakehata, MD[d], Livio Presutti, MD[a],
Domenico Villari, MD[a]

KEYWORDS

- Transcanal endoscopic approach • Cholesteatoma • Attic retraction
- Middle ear surgery • Residual • Recurrence

KEY POINTS

- Around the corner spaces can be easily visualized by endoscopic ear surgery.
- The surgical approach should respect as much as possible the physiology and the anatomy of the middle ear.
- Middle ear folds may play an important role in the blockage of ventilation routes, possibly provoking sectorial epitympanic dysventilation.
- Long-term results are crucial to validate a surgical technique to treat cholesteatoma.

INTRODUCTION

Surgical treatment of cholesteatoma remains controversial. Endoscopic instrumentation, techniques, and knowledge have improved over the last few years, and we believe that, in the future, endoscopic surgical techniques will gain increasing importance in otologic surgery. From our 9-year experience in endoscopic ear surgery, we believe that most of the spaces considered to be difficult to access with a microscopic technique could be visualized easily by endoscope-assisted surgery, and we believe that new anatomic concepts should be introduced for this. In this perspective, classic

The authors have no financial relationship to disclose.
[a] Otolaryngology Department, University Hospital of Modena, Via del Pozzo 71, Modena 41100, Italy; [b] Neurosurgery Department, New Civil Hospital Sant'Agostino-Estense, Stradello Baggiovara 53, Modena 41126, Italy; [c] Otolaryngology-Head and Neck Surgery Department, University Hospital of Verona, Piazzale Ludovico Antonio Scuro 10, Verona 37100, Italy; [d] Otolaryngology Department, University Hospital of Yamagata, 1-4-12 Kojirakawa-machi, Yamagata 990-8560, Japan
* Corresponding author. Otolaryngology Department, University Hospital of Modena, Via del Pozzo 71, Modena 41100, Italy.
E-mail address: matteo.alicandri@hotmail.it

Otolaryngol Clin N Am 49 (2016) 1265–1270
http://dx.doi.org/10.1016/j.otc.2016.05.015
0030-6665/16/$ – see front matter © 2016 Elsevier Inc. All rights reserved.

oto.theclinics.com

concepts of microscopic ear surgery, such as canal wall up and canal wall down tympanoplasties, could be completely modified on clinical and surgical practice.

When a new technique is introduced, it is essential to report results in the literature so the technique can be reviewed and hopefully accepted by scientific community. Because endoscopic ear surgery is a relatively new technique, few papers are present in the literature to report results.[1–3] The aim of present paper is to report the results at our institution (Modena University Hospitals) regarding endoscopic treatment of cholesteatoma at a mean follow-up of 5 years, so add to the experience reported previously on this topic.

MATERIAL AND METHODS

Starting in January 2006, we created a database in which all patients who underwent operation for middle ear indication and were followed in our clinic by regular visits at appropriate timing (in general after 1, 3, 6, and 12 months form the operation, then yearly) were included. At follow-up, patients were evaluated by an endoscopic office examination. Recurrences (defined as non–self-cleaning re-retraction of the attic requiring surgery) and residual (defined as insufficient primary resection of the epidermal matrix, presenting as cholesteatoma in absence of re-retraction of the tympanic membrane) were noted in the database. Residuals were defined by evaluations using computed tomography, performed most often at 1 year of follow-up or during a planned surgical second look. During September 2015, we reviewed the database to obtain results, and an analyses of 300 endoscopic or combined (endoscopic/microscopic) procedures to middle ear chronic otitis was performed. For the present study, only cholesteatomas treated endoscopically (exclusively or combined) with at least 3 years of follow-up were included for further analyses; canal wall down procedures were excluded.

RESULTS

The final study group included 244 ears (of 234 patients). The mean follow-up was 64.3 months (standard deviation 22.2). There were patients 166 (68%) free from disease during postoperative follow-up visit, 29 patients (12%) were diagnosed a recurrence, and 49 patients (20%) had residual disease (**Fig. 1**). Patients with

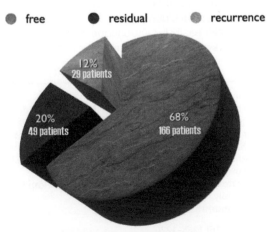

Fig. 1. Follow-up results. Blue color: free from disease; grey color: recurrence; red color: residual

recurrence and residual disease underwent second stage surgery and, in the final follow-up visit, another 50 patients (20.5%) were free from disease. There were 144 patients (69.5%) who underwent an exclusive endoscopic approach, whereas 100 patients (30.5%) underwent a combined approach with mastoidectomy (**Fig. 2**). Seventy-three patients (30%) had a cholesteatoma limited exclusively to the attic, whereas 44 (18%) had also a mesotympanic extension of the disease, 37 (15%) patients had an exclusive involvement of the mesotympanum, 73 (30%) had antral extension, and 17 (7%) had mastoid extension. There were 41 patients (17%) who were aged under 18 years, and 203 (83%) were adults.

In 45 patients (18.5%), it was possible to avoid ossicular removal, whereas in 199 patients (81.5%) ossicular removal and reconstruction was necessary (in these cases, an ossicular chain erosion or a infiltrative matrix of the medial aspect of the ossicles were found). There were 172 patients who underwent a cartilage reconstruction of the scutum (70%), in 36 patients the reconstruction was performed by bone (15%), and in 36 by (15%) temporalis fascia.

Based on our analyses and regarding age (>18 or <18 years old), a recurrence or residual was present in 68 adult patients (33%), and 10 recurrence or residual in 41 patients aged under 18 was noted (24%). Of 73 patients with cholesteatoma limited exclusively to the attic, 15 experienced residual disease; of 44 patients who also had a mesotympanic extension, 8 experienced residual pathology at follow-up, and of 37 patients with exclusive mesotympanic involvement, 5 experienced residual disease. Of 73 patients with antral extension, 18 experienced residual pathology, and of 17 patients with mastoid extension, 3 experienced residual pathology. Of 172 patients who underwent a cartilage reconstruction of the scutum, 19 experienced a recurrence; and of those 172, 36 underwent bone reconstruction of the scutum and 5 experienced a recurrence. Of those 172, 36 underwent a temporalis fascia reconstruction, and 5 experienced a recurrence.

DISCUSSION

Exclusive endoscopic tympanoplasty was first described by Tarabichi.[2] The new concept of endoscopic ear surgery redirected the attention away from the less critical areas (ie, mastoid) toward the tympanic cavity and its "hard-to-reach" extensions. The endoscopic technique was codified for a minimally invasive eradication of limited attic cholesteatoma, preserving the ossicular chain wherever possible with complete removal of the disease. From this indication, the clinical application of the transcanal

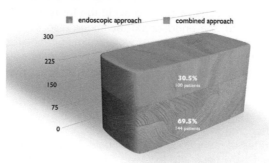

Fig. 2. Surgical approaches. Blue color: exclusive endoscopic approach; green color: combined approach.

endoscopic approach has allowed to extend the indication of this technique on the cholesteatoma of the whole tympanic cavity without mastoid involvement.

Primary acquired cholesteatoma is considered classically to be a manifestation of a retraction of the tympanic membrane that verifies when the sac advances into the tympanic cavity and to subsites such as the sinus tympani, the facial recess, the hypotympanum, and the attic.[4] In more advanced cases, a cholesteatoma progress further to reach the mastoid cavity. The main endpoints regarding results of operative intervention for cholesteatoma of the attic are the residual disease and recurrence. The residual disease is owing to an incomplete primary resection of the epidermal matrix, and presents a pearllike aspect. Insufficient resection may be owing an infiltrative epidermal matrix or to a limited exposition of hidden areas like the epitympanic space, retrotympanum, and sovratubal recess. Because the view during microscopic surgery is defined and limited by the narrowest segment of the ear canal, surgeons were forced to create a parallel port through the mastoid to gain keyhole access to the attic, although visualization with a microscope has proved to have distinct limitations. The surgeon can visualize structures only directly ahead and is unable to see objects that are "around the corner." So, this straightline view offered by the microscope resulted in certain blind pockets during middle ear surgery. These limitations can be overcome with the complementary help of an endoscope.[5] Thomassin and associates[6] found that, by using intraoperative endoscopy, the quality of disease eradication significantly improved and resulted in the dropping of the incidence of residual cholesteatoma from 47% to 6%. Youssef and Poe[7] found that the use of an endoscopic technique significantly decreased the morbidity of the second-look procedure, enhanced visualization of residual disease, and reduced operating time. Badr-El-Dine[8] reported on the value of endoscopy as an adjunct in cholesteatoma surgery and documented a reduced risk of residual when the endoscope was used. In the primary surgery after completion of microscopic cleaning, the overall incidence of intraoperative residuals detected with the endoscope was 22.8%; sinus tympani was the most common site of intraoperative residuals in both the canal wall up and canal wall down groups. At second-look endoscopic explorations, recurrences were identified in 8.6% of cases.

Recurrence consists in a new tympanic retraction pocket caused by inadequate reconstruction of the scutum and persistence of the physiopathologic process of middle ear depression. Although recurrence can be diagnosed otoscopically, residual cholesteatoma is classically independent of the eardrum and only surgical revision can determine definite diagnosis; this is the rationale for the second-look procedures, in addition to functional issues.[9] The persistence of physiopathologic phenomena that had determined the cholesteatoma development presents as a new attical retraction that requires a further surgical approach to avoid the formation of attical cholesteatoma again. In this regard, the endoscopic technique also helped to elucidate the pathophysiologic conditions that may provoke primary acquired cholesteatoma, and the selective epitmpanic dysventialtion syndrome was introduced.[10] By paying attention to ventilation routes blocks, the surgeon can restore physiologic conditions of airflow between mesotymanic spaces and epitympanic spaces, by opening or widening the epitymanic diaphragm, or by opening complete tensor folds, as previously.[11]

Because cholesteatoma is a chronic disease, with a possible long natural history and possibly high rates of recurrence and residuals, long-term results are crucial. In the literature, patients are generally followed for at least 5 years to assess failure rates.[12–15] In recent papers on this topic, report residual rates ranged from 3.5%[12] to 46%[13], whereas recurrence rates ranged from 2.8%[14] to 13%[15] at 5-years of follow-up. Unfortunately, papers dealing with cholesteatoma surgery are traditionally biased by heterogeneity of pathology, surgical techniques (ie, canal wall up, canal wall down, or others), low patient numbers, and doubts about methodology (ie, censorship); thus, the reported results are hardly comparable.

About the results of our study, as mentioned in Results, 165 patients (68%) were free from disease during postoperative follow-up visit, in 29 patients (12%) recurrence was diagnosed, and 49 patients (20%) had residual disease. Further experience and longer follow-up are necessary to confirm and clarify factors possibly influencing results. The long-term results of our cohort of patients are similar to those reported in the literature for microscopic surgery of cholesteatoma, especially regarding the recurrence rate. Two considerations must also be made. First, patients with longer follow-up in our cases series are those who were operated on at the beginning of the introduction of endoscopic technique in ear surgery. This could have influenced negatively the overall recurrence and residual rates. The second consideration is that, at least based on our data, results of endoscopic ear surgery are comparable in terms of residual pathology and recurrence to those of the literature, but endoscopic ear surgery allowed avoidance of most mastoidectomies, posterior tympanotomies, external incisions, and preservation of the ossicular chain. Being a minimally invasive approach, it eventually allowed to preserve ear structures as much as possible, with obvious benefits for patient quality of life.

SUMMARY

Endoscopic ear surgery can be considered an effective method to eradicate cholesteatoma from the middle ear. It provides better visualization of hidden areas and a better chance at tissue preservation. Minimally invasive access allows for a better understanding of the pathophysiology of cholesteatoma. Results can be compared with those reported for classic microscopic techniques in terms of recurrences or residual pathology at long-term follow-up. Further experiences, and even longer follow-up than reported are necessary to confirm our results.

REFERENCES

1. Migirov L, Shapira Y, Horowitz Z, et al. Exclusive endoscopic ear surgery for acquired cholesteatoma: preliminary results. Otol Neurotol 2011;32(3):433–6.
2. Tarabichi M. Endoscopic management of cholesteatoma: long-term results. Otolaryngol Head Neck Surg 2000;122(6):874–81.
3. Marchioni D, Villari D, Mattioli F, et al. Endoscopic management of attic cholesteatoma: a single-institution experience. Otolaryngol Clin North Am 2013;46(2):201–9.
4. Sheehy JL, Brackmann DE, Graham MD. Cholesteatoma surgery: residual and recurrent disease. A review of 1,024 cases. Ann Otol Rhinol Laryngol 1977;86:451–62.
5. Magnan J, Chays A, Lepetre C, et al. Surgical perspectives of endoscopy of the cerebellopontine angle. Am J Otol 1994;15:366–70.
6. Thomassin JM, Korchia D, Doris JM. Endoscopic-guided otosurgery in the prevention of residual cholesteatomas. Laryngoscope 1993;103:939–43.
7. Youssef TF, Poe DS. Endoscope-assisted second-stage tympanomastoidectomy. Laryngoscope 1997;107:1341–4.
8. Badr-el-Dine M. Value of ear endoscopy in cholesteatoma surgery. Otol Neurotol 2002;23:631–5.
9. Gaillardin L, Lescanne E, Morinière S, et al. Residual cholesteatoma: prevalence and location. Follow-up strategy in adults. Eur Ann Otorhinolaryngol Head Neck Dis 2012;129(3):136–40.

10. Marchioni D, Alicandri Ciufelli M, Molteni G, et al. Selective epitympanic dysventilation syndrome. Laryngoscope 2010;120:1028–33.
11. Marchioni D, Mattioli F, Alicandri-Ciufelli M, et al. Endoscopic evaluation of middle ear ventilation route blockage. Am J Otolaryngol 2010;31(6):453–66.
12. Trinidade A, Skingsley A, Yung MW. Mastoid obliteration surgery for cholesteatoma in 183 adult ears - a 5-year prospective cohort study. Clin Otolaryngol 2015;40(6):721–6.
13. Prasad SC, La Melia C, Medina M, et al. Long-term surgical and functional outcomes of the intact canal wall technique for middle ear cholesteatoma in the paediatric population [review]. Acta Otorhinolaryngol Ital 2014;34(5):354–61.
14. van Dinther JJ, Vercruysse JP, Camp S, et al. The bony obliteration tympanoplasty in pediatric cholesteatoma: long-term safety and hygienic results. Otol Neurotol 2015;36(9):1504–9.
15. Walker PC, Mowry SE, Hansen MR, et al. Long-term results of canal wall reconstruction tympanomastoidectomy. Otol Neurotol 2014;35(6):954–60.

Outcomes in Endoscopic Ear Surgery

Ruwan Kiringoda, MD, Elliott D. Kozin, MD, Daniel J. Lee, MD*

KEYWORDS

- Endoscopic ear surgery • EES • Transcanal endoscopic ear surgery • TEES
- Otoendoscopy • Outcomes • Cholesteatoma • Minimally invasive ear surgery

KEY POINTS

- Endoscopic ear surgery (EES) is an emerging surgical approach to manage complex middle ear and lateral skull base pathology.
- EES provides equivalent or improved rates of short-term and long-term control of chronic middle ear disease (cholesteatoma) compared with the microscope, while offering decreased morbidity of a minimally invasive approach.
- A growing number of noncholesteatoma otologic procedures are being performed endoscopically, with a wide spectrum of outcomes.
- Well-designed prospective studies on EES are needed to compare outcomes, morbidity, and cost utility compared with microscopic approaches.

INTRODUCTION

Endoscopic ear surgery (EES) provides several advantages compared with traditional surgical microscopy. Rigid endoscopy allows for wide-field view of the surgical field, improved resolution with high magnification, and the ability to "look around corners," enabling direct visualization of the hidden recesses, including the retrotympanum, epitympanum, supratubal recess, protympanum, and hypotympanum.

Endoscopic visualization of the middle ear was first described in the 1960s.[1] Advances in endoscopic instrumentation and video technology allowed Poe and colleagues[2] to describe the use of small-diameter endoscopes to explore the middle ear through a strategically placed myringotomy in the early 1990s. Later that decade, Muaaz Tarabichi described middle ear surgery performed exclusively via endoscopic visualization.[3–5] Modern high-definition video systems now provide superior image quality that has made endoscopic middle ear surgery a viable alternative to the microscopic techniques in several centers in the United States and abroad (**Fig. 1**), but there

Disclosure Statement: The authors have nothing to disclose.
Department of Otology and Laryngology, Massachusetts Eye and Ear Infirmary, Harvard Medical School, 243 Charles Street, Boston, MA 02114, USA
* Corresponding author.
E-mail address: Daniel_Lee@meei.harvard.edu

Otolaryngol Clin N Am 49 (2016) 1271–1290
http://dx.doi.org/10.1016/j.otc.2016.05.008
0030-6665/16/$ – see front matter © 2016 Elsevier Inc. All rights reserved.

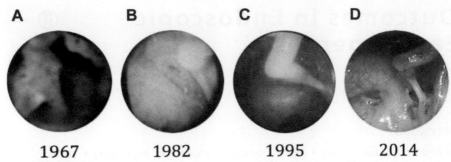

1967   1982   1995   2014

Fig. 1. Endoscopic images of the left middle ear: a timeline. The evolution of endoscopic and video technologies, especially over the past 2 decades, has led to significant progress in endoscopic visualization of the middle ear and have paved the way for EES. (A) 1967: Mer and colleagues endoscopic view of the stapes. The development of coherent fiberoptic bundles for image transmission, and an incoherent bundle for light transmission by Hopkins facilitated the development of otoendoscopes. (B) 1982: Nomura and colleagues demonstrate angled endoscopy of middle ear feasible using a 2.2 mm diameter "needle otoscope." (C) 1995: Image from the first US otoendoscopy and temporal bone dissection course manual. (D) 2014: High resolution image from modern 0° 3 mm rigid otoendoscope. (From [A] Mer SB, Derbyshire AJ, Brushenko A, et al. Fiberoptic endotoscopes for examining the middle ear. Arch Otolaryngol 1967;85(4):387–93, with permission; [B] Nomura Y. Effective photography in otolaryngology-head and neck surgery: endoscopic photography of the middle ear. Otolaryngol Head Neck Surg 1982;90(4):397, with permission; [C] From Poe D. Otoendoscopy and temporal bone dissection - a course manual. St Louis (MO): St Louis University, 1995; and [D] Courtesy of Daniel Lee, MD, Boston, MA.)

has been slow adoption of EES due to good outcomes with traditional techniques, lack of EES exposure during residency and fellowship training, limited instrumentation, and concerns about one handed surgery and poor depth perception.

A similar reluctance to adopt endoscopic techniques in otolaryngology was seen with the introduction of the endoscope for sinus surgery in the 1980s and 1990s. Opponents expressed similar concerns about the endoscopic compared with microscopic sinus surgery approaches. Nevertheless, the endoscope today represents the gold standard for the management of sinus disease, based on advantages that include improved visualization, decreased blood loss, and better access to pathology while avoiding transfacial and/or sublabial incisions.[6,7]

A slowly growing body of literature (particularly from centers outside the United States) over the past two decades describes expanding roles for EES. Currently, binocular microscopy remains gold standard. Traditional microscopic approaches provide the benefits of two-handed dissection and depth perception offered by binocular vision (despite the possible need for increased drilling and tissue retraction) and greater proficiency by most surgeons associated with adequate exposure during training. In contrast, proponents of EES suggest several distinct advantages over the microscope, such as improved visualization and access to the hidden recesses of the middle ear, avoidance of a postauricular incision in many cases, and less bony drilling. In ideal form, this minimally invasive approach holds the promise of decreased operative time, less postoperative morbidity, and diminished need for mastoidectomy surgery. In this review, we seek to evaluate the current body of literature regarding EES outcomes, review our EES outcomes at the Massachusetts Eye and Ear Infirmary (MEEI), and compare these results with published data for microscopic surgery.

Appropriate classification of techniques used during otologic surgery is prerequisite to accurately categorizing outcomes. We differentiate between *observational EES*, which involves endoscopic inspection (otoendoscopy) during an otherwise microscope-only procedure, and *operative EES*, which ranges from mixed dissection with endoscopic and microscopic techniques, to a transcanal endoscope-only surgical technique. Accordingly, at MEEI we use an EES classification system for documentation purposes that ranges from 0 (microscope-only case) to 3 (transcanal endoscopic ear surgery, TEES; **Table 1**).[8] We define TEES as middle ear surgery performed entirely using the endoscope for visualization, without the use of the operating microscope. Finally, we define residual disease as hidden cholesteatoma that remains and is detected during primary surgery with the endoscope following microscopic resection or identified at a second-look procedure. Recurrence of disease is defined as cholesteatoma formation from a new retraction pocket.

The most widely studied application of EES is for management of cholesteatoma. This indication exploits the biggest advantage of the endoscope: the ability to look around corners when using a transcanal approach without depending on line-of-sight surgery needed when using the binocular microscope. We seek to quantify disease control through a comparison of residual/recurrent disease. Additionally, we seek to further highlight other applications of EES, including myringoplasty, tympanoplasty, ossiculoplasty, and relevant hearing outcomes, as well as describe outcomes with other otologic procedures, such as cochlear implantation, stapedectomy, and approaches to the lateral skull base.

In this review, we aim to comprehensively review observational and operational EES outcomes. We further aim to compare EES outcomes with data from microscopic procedures. We hypothesize that EES is a reasonable and less invasive approach compared with microscopic techniques for the management of routine and complex otologic disease.

OBSERVATIONAL ENDOSCOPIC EAR SURGERY FOR CHOLESTEATOMA: ANALYSIS OF OUTCOMES

Observational EES refers to the use of endoscopes for visualization only and as an adjunct to the operating microscope. **Table 2** shows outcomes associated with observational endoscopic cholesteatoma resection. Articles range from 10 to 294 patients, and follow-up duration ranges from 3 months to 12 years.

Particularly salient are direct comparisons of endoscopic and microscopic techniques. In one of the largest series, Badr-El-Dine[9] used endoscopic observation following the completion of microscopic canal wall up (CWU) and canal wall down (CWD) procedures; they discovered the prevalence of residual disease missed by

Table 1				
Massachusetts Eye and Ear Infirmary EES classification system				
	Class 0	Class 1	Class 2	Class 3
Intraoperative use of endoscope	None	Inspection only	Mixed dissection	Endoscope only
	Microscope-only case	Endoscope used to assess disease	Microscope and endoscope used for dissection	No use of microscope
	Non-TEES			TEES

Abbreviations: EES, endoscopic ear surgery; TEES, transcanal endoscopic ear surgery.

Table 2
Use of endoscopes predominantly for observation in cholesteatoma procedures

Authors	Study Design	1st Procedures	Residual at 1st Procedure	Mean Follow-up (Range)	Cholesteatoma Found During Second Look	Pediatric Patients
Thomassin et al,[53] 1993	Group A: microscope alone; group B: microscope + endoscopy. Second look with endoscope in all cases	Group A = 36 Group B = 44	N/A	N/A (12–18 mo)	Group A = 47.7% (n = 21); Group B = 5.5% (n = 2)	Yes (n = 20)
Rosenberg et al,[21] 1995	Endoscope for second look, then microscopic confirmation	10	N/A	N/A (8 mo–9 y)	50.0% (n = 5)	Yes (n = 10)
Youssef & Poe,[54] 1997	Endoscope for second look, then microscopic confirmation	13	N/A	N/A (6–12 mo)	23.1% (n = 3)	Yes (n = 5)
Haberkamp & Tanyeri,[55] 1999	Endoscope for second look, then microscopic confirmation	15	N/A	N/A	Endoscope 20.0% (n = 1); microscope 50% (n = 5)	Unknown
Good & Isaacson,[22] 1999	Endoscope as microscope adjunct during 1st procedure; second-look only performed in select patients	29	24.1% (n = 7)	6.4 mo (12–18 mo)	18.2% (n = 2 of 11)	Yes (n = 29)
Badr-El-Dine,[56] 2002	Endoscope as microscope adjunct during 1st procedure; second look with endoscope for both observation and dissection	92	22.8% (n = 21)	N/A (9–12 mo)	8.6% (n = 3 of 35)	Unknown
El-Meselaty et al,[57] 2003	Group A: Endoscope used as microscope adjunct during primary procedure for observation and dissection; group B: primary procedure performed with microscope alone; Second look with endoscope for observation and dissection	Group A = 40 Group B = 42	Group A = 40.0% (n = 16)	14.5 mo (12–18 mo)	Group A = 0% (n = 0 of 5); Group B = 42.9% (n = 3 of 7)	Yes

Study	Procedure	N	Second look	Follow-up	Residual disease	Improved access/visualization
Ayache et al,[58] 2008	Group A: primary procedure performed with microscope alone; group B: endoscope as microscope adjunct during primary procedure for observation and dissection	Group A = 157 Group B = 80	Group B = 44% (n = 35)	N/A	37.5% (n = 6 of 16)	Yes
Presutti et al,[59] 2008	Endoscope as microscope adjunct during primary procedure for observation and dissection; second look performed in select patients	32	37.5% (n = 12)	34 mo (N/A)	16.7% (2 of 12)	Unknown
Badr-El-Dine,[9] 2009	Endoscope as microscope adjunct during primary procedure for observation and dissection; second look performed in select patients	294	16.7% (n = 49)	28.2 mo (N/A)	8.6% (n = 8 of 93)	Unknown
Sarcu & Isaacson,[11] 2015	Endoscopy used for inspection following microscopic resection of disease	42	17% (n = 7)	N/A	42% in 12 high-risk patients who had second looks	Yes
Farahani et al,[10] 2015	Endoscopy used for inspection following tympanomeatal flap elevation and following microscopic resection of disease	58 (13 with Cholesteatoma)	31% (n = 4)	N/A	N/A - no second look performed	

Abbreviation: N/A, not applicable.
Adapted from Kozin ED, Gulati S, Kaplan AB, et al. Systematic review of outcomes following observational and operative endoscopic middle ear surgery. Laryngoscope 2015;125(5):1205–14; with permission.

the microscope, but detected with the endoscope, was 16.7%. Residual disease was most frequently found in regions where line of sight limitations preclude direct microscopic visualization, while the endoscopic view remains intact: the sinus tympani was the most common site of residual disease in both CWU and CWD groups (36.7%), followed by the facial recess (28.6%), the undersurface of the scutum in the CWU cases (20.4%), and the anterior epitympanic recess (14.3%).

Farahani and colleagues[10] prospectively compared microscopic and endoscopic modalities via a cohort study of 58 patients with chronic otitis media who underwent a microscopic postauricular tympanoplasty with or without mastoidectomy. After a tympanomeatal flap was elevated, the middle ear was evaluated, and the investigators found that the epitympanic, posterior mesotympanic (retrotympanic), and hypotympanic structures were better visualized endoscopically. Moreover, 14 patients with cholesteatoma underwent microscope-only resection, followed by endoscopic reevaluation at the conclusion of the case, which revealed residual disease in 31% (n = 4) of patients. In similar fashion, Sarcu and Isaacson performed otoendoscopy on 42 patients at the conclusion of microscopic resection of cholesteatoma and found 17% with residual disease.[11]

Overall, the summary and comparison data suggest that the enhanced visualization and ability to visualize difficult-to-see regions of the middle ear make observational endoscopic techniques a valuable adjunct to improve outcomes yielded by traditional microscopic techniques.

OPERATIVE ENDOSCOPIC EAR SURGERY/TRANSCANAL ENDOSCOPIC EAR SURGERY FOR CHOLESTEATOMA: ANALYSIS OF OUTCOMES

Overall rates of recurrent and residual disease following traditional microscopic surgical mastoidectomy procedures are well studied. Large analyses show residual disease in 10% to 40% of ears following CWU tympanomastoidectomy.[12–14] CWD procedures offer significantly lower risk of residual disease at a cost of greater morbidity: patients undergoing these procedures require lifelong maintenance of the mastoid bowl, while facing persistent issues with thermal sensitivity, caloric stimulation, water precautions, and cosmetic alterations of the meatus.[15,16]

Performing mixed or fully endoscopic dissection (operative EES) gives the advantages of decreased rates of residual disease associated with observational EES, while potentially avoiding the sequelae of postauricular incision and mastoidectomy. **Table 3** lists findings from publications describing EES classified as MEEI class 1 to 3. The number of procedures ranges from 12 to 184, and follow-up ranges from 16 months to 11 years. Importantly, the conversion from TEES to microscopic surgery occurred in 4.3% to 23.8% of procedures, suggesting that most procedures started with a transcanal endoscopic approach can be completed without the need for conversion to the operating microscope. Noted complications include a single case of delayed facial palsy, as well as several cases of postoperative tympanic membrane (TM) perforation, graft lateralization, and decrease in sensorineural hearing. No major complications, such as permanent facial nerve injury or profound sensorineural hearing loss were noted.

With respect to cholesteatoma control, Presutti and colleagues[17] performed a systematic review examining data from 7 independent studies to compare residual and recurrent disease following EES relative to established open techniques. A cumulative analysis of 515 patients who underwent 517 surgeries (57% TEES, 43% combined technique including mastoidectomy) showed 32 patients (6.2%) with

Table 3
Operative endoscopic ear surgery in cholesteatoma surgery, including transcanal endoscopic ear surgery

Authors	n*	Mean Follow-up (Range)	Second Look/ Revisions	Residual Cholesteatoma on Second Look	Conversion to Microscope?	Hearing Outcomes?	Pediatric Patients?	Complications
Yung,[60] 1994	92	N/A	N/A	N/A	Case started with microscope	N/A	Unknown	N/A
Bottrill & Poe,[61] 1995	14	7 (6–12 mo)	Yes	3 of 9 (33.3%)	Yes (n = 2 for 1° procedure; n = 2 for 2° procedure)	N/A	Yes	No
Tarabichi,[3] 1997	36	41 mo (N/A)	Yes	n = 4 (unknown %)	No	Yes	Yes	Tympanic membrane defect (n = 9), 15 dB worsened bone conduction at 3000 Hz (n = 1)
Tarabichi,[5] 2000	69	41 mo (N/A)	Yes (n = 6)	Unknown	Yes (4.3%, n = 3)	Yes	Unknown	15 dB worsened bone conduction at 3000 Hz (n = 1)
Yung,[62] 2001	231	N/A (1–12 y)	Yes	19 of 231 (8.2%)	Case started with microscope	N/A	Yes	N/A
Tarabichi,[63] 2004	73	43 mo (N/A)	Yes	n = 6 (Unknown %)	No	Yes	Yes	N/A
Barakate & Bottrill,[13] 2008	68	16 mo (N/A)	Yes	14 of 68 (20.6%)	Yes (5.9%, n = 4)	N/A	Yes	N/A

(continued on next page)

Table 3
(continued)

Authors	n*	Mean Follow-up (Range)	Second Look/Revisions	Residual Cholesteatoma on Second Look	Conversion to Microscope?	Hearing Outcomes?	Pediatric Patients?	Complications
Marchioni et al,[64] 2009	21	23 mo (N/A)	No	N/A	Yes (23.8%, n = 5)	Yes	Unknown	No
Migirov et al,[65] 2011	30	N/A (0–1 y)	No	N/A	No	Yes	Yes	Worsening of sensorineural hearing loss (n = 2)
Marchioni et al,[66] 2011	68	18 (6–48) mo	Yes	3 of 23 (13.0%)	No	No	Unknown	No
Marchioni et al,[67] 2013	146	31.2 mo (N/A)	Yes	11 of 46 (7.5%)	Yes (17.8%, n = 26)	No	Yes	N/A
Hanna et al,[68] 2014	184	3.2 (1–11) y	Yes	86 of 184	Yes—combined approach	Yes	Yes	N/A
Cohen et al,[8] 2016	121 (55 chole)	N/A	Yes	9 of 25 (36%)	Yes—51 TEES, 70 mixed dissection	Yes	Yes	N/A
Marchioni et al,[23] 2015	31	36 (8–88) mo	Yes	10 of 31 (32.2%)	No—31 TEES compared to 28 CWU control	Yes	Yes	Delayed facial palsy (n = 1), TM lateralization (N = 1)
Kobayashi et al,[24] 2015	12	23.1 (3–51) mo	Yes	1 of 1 (100%)	No	Yes	Yes	Temporary tympanic membrane defect (n = 2)

Abbreviations: chole, cholesteatoma; CWU, canal wall up; n*, number of procedures; TM, tympanic membrane; TEES, transcanal endoscopic ear surgery.

Adapted from Kozin ED, Gulati S, Kaplan AB, et al. Systematic review of outcomes following observational and operative endoscopic middle ear surgery. Laryngoscope 2015;125(5):1205–14; with permission.

residual and 16 patients (3.1%) with recurrent cholesteatoma, with a mean follow-up of 23.4 months. The overall results of TEES in conjunction with selected EES/microscopic approaches compare favorably with established results for open CWU techniques. Although longer duration of follow-up is needed, endoscopic technique appears to be associated with superior control of middle ear disease and reduction in the number of mastoidectomies.

Several studies examined hearing outcomes following cholesteatoma removal. Marchioni and colleagues compared 31 TEES procedures with 28 microscopic CWU controls, noting similar pure tone average outcomes following both TEES and microscopic placement of partial and total ossicular replacement prostheses (PORPs and TORPs.) In addition, they found that ossicular chain preservation was statistically more likely in TEES (42%) than in microscopic CWU (10%) surgery, and these patients had the best postoperative hearing outcomes. The remaining studies reviewed provide predominantly descriptive outcomes following endoscopic PORP and TORP placed during cholesteatoma surgery, suggesting that although ossicular chain reconstruction can be performed, additional comparative outcome data are needed to better quantify outcomes following microscopic versus endoscopic procedures.

ENDOSCOPIC EAR SURGERY FOR PEDIATRIC CHOLESTEATOMA

Cholesteatoma in children is characterized by more aggressive growth, more infiltrative disease, and higher rates of recidivism compared with adults.[18–20] Many of the articles reviewed in **Tables 2–4** incorporate a mixed pediatric and adult population, but do not stratify outcomes on age, but several articles focus exclusively on pediatric chronic ear disease.[11,21–24] Most pertinently, Cohen, Lee, and colleagues at MEEI demonstrated an average residual rate of 36% after primary endoscopic cholesteatoma resection followed by planned endoscopic second look, which compares favorably with non-EES pediatric outcomes, that range from 5% to 71%.[8,25] Operative times and rates of tympanoplasty closure were examined and found to be similar, whereas the TEES group demonstrated superior audiometric outcomes.[8]

Marchioni and colleagues[23] compared 31 ears in pediatric patients undergoing TEES with 28 patients who underwent microscopic CWU tympanomastoidectomy for cholesteatoma; Residual disease was lower (19.3%) for TEES than for the microscopic group (34.4%) and Kaplan-Meier analysis at 36 months showed a lower recurrence rate for the TEES group; however, the small number of patients prevented either result from reaching statistical significance.

Kobayashi and colleagues[24] describe their experience with congenital cholesteatoma (CC) and TEES. Twelve children with CC confined to the middle ear underwent TEES. No surgical complications were noted. Over a mean follow-up of 23 (range 3–51) months, 1 of 12 patients (8.3%) was noted to have residual cholesteatoma on a planned second-look procedure, and the other 11 patients showed no evidence of residual disease. This compares favorably with traditional microscopic techniques, which range from 10.5% to 45.5%.[26,27]

The benefits of EES for pediatric patients are potentially numerous; in addition to control of aggressive disease, there is greater impetus to avoid CWD surgery, obviating the need for repeated cleanings, aggressive dry ear precautions, and lifestyle changes in childhood as a consequence of an open mastoid cavity. As a result, many surgeons favor canal-wall sparing procedures, and second looks are performed routinely for pediatric cholesteatoma. EES offers significant potential utility for control

Table 4
Operative endoscopic ear surgery for myringoplasty, tympanoplasty, ossiculoplasty

Publication	Indication	n*	Mean Follow-Up (Range)	Use of Microscope	Major Finding	Complication	Pediatric Patients
el-Guindy,[69] 1992	Myringoplasty	36	N/A (1.5–6 mo)	No	Graft take rate was 91.7% (n = 33) and the air-bone gap was closed to <10 dB in 83.3% (n = 30)	NA	No
Tarabichi,[4] 1999	Several	165	Varies by indication	No	Transcanal approach was used without conversion to postauricular open approach in all tympanoplasty procedures (n = 96) and 50 of 53 procedures performed for acquired cholesteatoma	Worsening bone conduction (15 dB at 3 kHz) (n = 1), blunting of anterior sulcus, TM cholesteatoma pearl formation (n = 1)	Yes
Usami et al,[70] 2001	Myringoplasty	22	24.5 (6–36) mo	No	Closure of the perforation was seen in 18 of 22 ears; reduced air-bone gaps were seen in all ears	N/A	Yes
Jang et al,[71] 2006	Cranular myringitis	21	11 (3–2.6 y) mo	No	18 of 21 patients were cured after a single treatment, 3 of 21 required multiple treatments; no recurrences observed during follow-up	N/A	Unknown
Kakehata et al,[72] 2006	Ossiculoplasty	9	17 (7–24) mo	No	Average hearing level improved from 59 dB to 27 dB postsurgically, with an average air-bone gap of 11 dB	Inserted cartilage bent (n = 1)	Yes
Yadav et al,[73] 2009	Myringoplasty	50	8 wk (N/A)	No	Successful graft uptake in 80% of patients; of these patients, air-bone gap showed a >20 dB improvement in 1 patient, 11–20 dB improvement in 30 patients, and 0–10 dB improvement in 9 patients	N/A	No

Study	Procedure	n*	Follow-up		Outcomes	Complications	
Marchioni et al,[74] 2010	Several	27	20.1 mo (N/A)	Yes	5 patients received microscopic meatoplasty before transcanal approach; mastoid bone was preserved in all 21 of 27 patients with no recurrence of disease at follow-up	N/A	Unknown
Konstantinidis et al,[75] 2013	Myringoplasty	82	N/A (0–6 mo)	No	Closure of the perforation was seen in 85.4% of patients; closure rate decreased when the size of the perforation was >30% of the pars tensa	N/A	No
Ayache,[28] 2013	Myringoplasty	30	N/A (2–12 mo)	Yes	Preoperative microscope revealed total exposure in 27% of cases vs 100% of endoscope cases; 96% of patients had a closed perforation at 1 y follow-up	Iatrogenic cholesteatoma in TM (n = 2)	Yes
Marchioni et al,[76] 2013	Several	6	8.5 (5–18) mo	No	Exclusive endoscopic transcanal approach used in all patients; no pathology recurrence at follow-up	N/A	No
Furukawa et al,[29] 2014	Myringoplasty	25	9.8 (5–18) mo	Yes	Greater visualization of the tympanic membrane and perforation edges with the endoscope (25/25) as compared with the microscope (20/25)	N/A	Yes

Abbreviations: n*, number of procedures; N/A, not applicable; TM, tympanic membrane.

Adapted from Kozin ED, Gulati S, Kaplan AB, et al. Systematic review of outcomes following observational and operative endoscopic middle ear surgery. Laryngoscope 2015;125(5):1205–14; with permission.

of disease as well as avoidance of mastoid surgery during both primary surgery and second-look approaches.

ENDOSCOPIC MYRINGOPLASTY, TYMPANOPLASTY, OSSICULOPLASTY

Endoscopic myringoplasty, tympanoplasty, and ossiculoplasty performed independently of cholesteatoma surgery are summarized in **Table 4**. Studies range from 9 to 165 patients, and most are characterized by an exclusive transcanal endoscopic approach (MEEI class 3). Hearing improvement with ossiculoplasty is consistently demonstrated, although no large studies systematically compare endoscopic and microscopic techniques. Rates of perforation closure vary greatly across studies, and visualization of the entire perforation is more consistently achieved endoscopically than microscopically.[28,29] Although conclusive data are limited, the full range of tympanoplasty procedures, including lateral graft tympanoplasty, can be performed endoscopically.[30]

The utility of EES for stapes surgery is controversial, as the microscope provides excellent outcomes. Although the endoscope provides excellent visualization and rapid assessment of the footplate, facial nerve, and round window, bone removal is still needed as current instrumentation and laser handpieces are currently designed for line-of-sight surgery.

A retrospective series of 20 patients following endoscopic stapedectomy showed adequate exposure of the footplate in 95% of cases. Postoperative audiometry demonstrated complete air-bone gap closure in 55%, mild conductive hearing loss (up to 20 dB) in 30%, and mixed hearing loss in 2 cases. No other major complications were observed, leading the investigators to conclude that the procedure is safe and outcomes are acceptable.[31] A recent prospective study comparing 15 endoscopic and 41 microscopic procedures found no differences of operating time or postoperative hearing ouctomes.[32] Daneshi and Jahandideh[33] performed a similar comparison between 19 endoscopic and 15 microscopic stapedectomies and, in addition to similar audiometric outcomes between groups, found that endoscopic surgery was associated with greater patient comfort and allowed for the elimination of ear canal packing at the conclusion of the procedure. More prospective studies examining outcomes with endoscopic stapedectomy are needed. As endoscopic dissection around the footplate can be technically challenging, this approach should be performed only by the most experienced EES surgeons.

ENDOSCOPIC COCHLEAR IMPLANTATION

Cochlear implantation (CI) represents a more recent and controversial application of EES. Operative endoscopy permits transcanal access and magnified visualization of the round window. **Table 5** summarizes the results of several small studies (between 5 and 13 patients) featuring patients who underwent endoscopic CI.[34–36] Overall, complete round window insertions were achieved in nearly all patients via a mastoidectomy-sparing suprameatal approach; no major noted perioperative or postoperative complications, although follow-up duration is limited. Despite the allure of these results, caution is advised. Tarabichi and colleagues[37] assessed orientation of the basal turn of the cochlear in 100 temporal bone computed tomography scans and concluded that the trajectory provided by posterior tympanotomy aligns more favorably with the basal turn of the cochlea than the transcanal access afforded by EES. For this reason, a traditional CWU mastoidectomy with facial recess remains favored for CI.

Table 5
Endoscopic cochlear implantation

Publication	Indication	n*	Mean Follow-Up (Range)	Use of Microscope	Major Finding	Complication	Pediatric Patients?
Migirov et al,[36] 2015	Cochlear implant	13	N/A (0–4 y)	No	Complete electrode insertion via the round window was achieved and the chorda tympani nerve was preserved in all cases	N/A	Yes
Marchioni et al,[34] 2014	Cochlear implant	6	7.3 (1–11) mo	No	In 5 of 6 patients, the endoscopic cochlear implant was placed without complications	Chorda tympani injury (n = 1)	No
Marchioni et al,[35] 2015	Cochlear implant	5	6 (4–12) mo	No	In 5 of 8 patients with anomalous middle ear anatomy, the endoscopic cochlear implant was placed without complications	None	Yes

Abbreviation: n*, number of procedures.

Adapted from Kozin ED, Gulati S, Kaplan AB, et al. Systematic review of outcomes following observational and operative endoscopic middle ear surgery. Laryngoscope 2015;125(5):1205–14; with permission.

ENDOSCOPIC SKULL BASE SURGERY

Endoscopic visualization also can be used to facilitate lateral skull base procedures, including approaches to the internal auditory canal (IAC) or petrous apex. Cadaveric studies have demonstrated utility during approaches to the skull base, such as the demonstration of keyhole craniotomy in for tumor dissection in the IAC, endoscopic identification of the posterior semicircular canal during retrosigmoid approaches, or transcanal endoscopic cochlea-sparing approaches to the IAC, as described by our group at MEEI and others.[38–40]

Wackym and colleagues[41] initially described the use of the endoscope during vestibular schwannoma surgery to identify residual tumor (particularly in the fundus) and exposed air cells in the decompressed internal auditory canal that were not appreciated microscopically. Additional studies have shown efficacy of skull base endoscopy for identification of cranial nerve anatomy as well as removal of residual tumor undetected by the microscope.[42,43] Most recently, Kumon and colleagues,[44] in a prospective study, demonstrated a lower rate of residual tumor in 28 patients who underwent combined endoscopic/microsurgical resection, as compared with 43 patients who underwent microsurgical resection alone.

Innovative work by Presutti, Alicandri-Ciufelli, and colleagues[45,46] in Italy has explored the use of the endoscope for transcanal lateral skull base surgery. Indications include cochlear schwannoma or disease in the petrous apex. Marchioni and colleagues[47] provide the most in-depth description of endoscopic skull base surgeries, delineating a series of successful transcanal approaches to address pathology involving the fundus, IAC, cochlea, petrous apex, and geniculate ganglion region, with no major postoperative adverse outcomes. Currently, outcomes are essentially limited to case reports and small retrospective series. Additional refinement of this technique, along with more extensive retrospective and prospective studies, are needed to better understand the role of the endoscope for minimally invasive lateral skull base surgery.

At MEEI, otologic endoscopy is also used as an adjunct in open lateral skull base procedures, such as vestibular schwannoma resection and auditory brainstem implantation (ABI). Following a traditional suboccipital tumor resection, endoscopic visualization is used to identify any air cells tracts originating in the internal auditory canal to allow for application of surgical wax to prevent cerebrospinal fluid leak. During ABI, endoscopic visualization provides a detailed view of brainstem anatomy, which facilitates placement of the ABI leads at the appropriate auditory sites in the brainstem. Surgical endoscopy is also used for visualization of the superior semicircular canal during middle fossa repair of canal dehiscence.[48] Studies are ongoing to better describe and quantify the effects of the endoscope on relevant outcomes.

ENDOSCOPIC EAR SURGERY AT MASSACHUSETTS EYE AND EAR INFIRMARY

At MEEI, transcanal endoscopic middle ear surgery was first started by the senior author (DJL) in 2012. From 2012 through 2014, a total of 448 EES cases were performed, including 220 pediatric and 228 adult cases. The introduction of the endoscope has influence the number of CWD mastoidectomies for primary cholesteatoma, from 5.9% in 2011 to 0.35% in 2014 (**Table 6**). We are performing a retrospective review of our pediatric and adult EES outcomes for the first 3 years and will begin a prospective study comparing EES with microscopic techniques in 2016.

Table 6			
Endoscopic ear surgery has reduced the number of canal wall down (CWD) mastoidectomies for primary cholesteatoma			
Year	Total Number of Cases	Number of CWD Cases for Primary Cholesteatoma	% CWD Cases
2010	185	5	2.7
2011	170	19	5.9
2012	218	8	3.7
2013	265	1	0.4
2014	285	1	0.35

Total number of cases includes all chronic ear procedures including cholesteatoma, ossicular chain reconstruction, and tympanoplasty before and after the introduction of EES in 2012. Revision CWD cases excluded.

NEED FOR PROSPECTIVE AND SAFETY STUDIES

To date, there have been no large, documented, prospective trials comparing TEES to traditional microscopic surgery. Our prospective trial at MEEI will focus on surgical outcomes (residual/recurrent disease, need for reoperation, audiometric outcomes, complications), perioperative considerations (operating time, procedures performed, conversion from TEES to microscopic approach, need for postauricular incision and/or mastoidectomy), and patient-centered outcomes (objective measures of postoperative pain, disability, pain medication needs, surgical site morbidity, postauricular/periauricular hypesthesia). **Table 7** represents our considerations for critical outcome variables in designing a comprehensive prospective trial of TEES.

Although many of the cited works address surgical efficacy, there is minimal available data regarding differences in pain, morbidity, postoperative recovery, and other relevant perioperative and patient-centered variables. A comprehensive perioperative evaluation is needed to quantify the benefits of EES.

Studies at MEEI and elsewhere have explored safety considerations unique to EES, such as the effects of radiant exposure on temperature changes in the middle ear, or evaluating the potential ototoxicity of defog solution.[49–52] Undoubtedly, additional safety considerations unique to EES will emerge.

Table 7		
Outcome measures for prospective trials of endoscopic ear surgery		
Perioperative Considerations	Surgical Outcomes	Patient-centered Outcomes
Radiologic classification of disease	Residual/recurrent disease	Postoperative pain/disability
Surgical approach with MEEI EES classification	Audiometric outcomes	Pain medication requirements
Operative times	Need for reoperation	Surgical site morbidity
Need for postauricular incision	Complications	Post/periauricular hypesthesia
Need for mastoidectomy		

Abbreviations: EES, endoscopic ear surgery; MEEI, Massachusetts Eye and Ear Infirmary.

SUMMARY

The spectrum of EES is growing in scope and frequency of use, while being applied to a broad range of middle ear and skull base pathologies. Current data suggest that EES provides equivalent short-term and long-term control of chronic middle ear disease (cholesteatoma) compared with microscopic approaches, while offering the potentially decreased morbidity of a minimally invasive approach. Outcomes following tympanoplasty, ossiculoplasty, and stapedectomy are also promising in terms of delivering equivalent hearing outcomes via an endoscopic approach. Despite a rapidly growing collection of retrospective analyses and case series, there remains a distinct lack of large prospective studies to better evaluate the short-term and long-term outcomes of EES in relation to the gold standard of surgical microscopy, as well as patient-centered outcome studies that can quantify benefit of minimally invasive surgery. Additional retrospective and prospective studies are needed to further classify the efficacy and presumed reduced morbidity of endoscopic middle ear surgery.

The role of the endoscope beyond tympanoplasty/mastoidectomy surgery is still evolving. A number of smaller studies suggest that the endoscope can be a valuable adjunct during vestibular schwannoma resection and approaches to the petrous apex, and anatomic studies of transcanal endoscopic corridors to the skull base suggest that endoscopy may play an enlarging role in lateral skull base surgery. Additional studies and refinement of operative techniques will be critical to these applications of EES in the future.

REFERENCES

1. Mer SB, Derbyshire AJ, Brushenko A, et al. Fiberoptic endotoscopes for examining the middle ear. Arch Otolaryngol 1967;85(4):387–93.
2. Poe DS, Rebeiz EE, Pankratov MM, et al. Transtympanic endoscopy of the middle ear. Laryngoscope 1992;102(9):993–6.
3. Tarabichi M. Endoscopic management of acquired cholesteatoma. Am J Otol 1997;18(5):544–9.
4. Tarabichi M. Endoscopic middle ear surgery. Ann Otol Rhinol Laryngol 1999; 108(1):39–46.
5. Tarabichi M. Endoscopic management of cholesteatoma: long-term results. Otolaryngol Head Neck Surg 2000;122(6):874–81.
6. Vining EM, Kennedy DW. The transmigration of endoscopic sinus surgery from Europe to the United States. Ear Nose Throat J 1994;73(7):456–8, 460.
7. Chandra RK, Conley DB, Kern RC. Evolution of the endoscope and endoscopic sinus surgery. Otolaryngol Clin North Am 2009;42(5):747–52, vii.
8. Cohen MS, Landegger LD, Kozin ED, et al. Pediatric endoscopic ear surgery in clinical practice: lessons learned and early outcomes. Laryngoscope 2016; 126(3):732–8.
9. Badr-el-Dine M. Surgery of sinus tympani cholesteatoma: endoscopic necessity. J Int Adv Otol 2009;5:158–65.
10. Farahani F, Shariatpanahi E, Jahanshahi J, et al. Diagnostic performance of endoscopic and microscopic procedures for identifying different middle ear structures and remaining disease in patients with chronic otitis media: a prospective cohort study. PLoS One 2015;10(7):e0132890.
11. Sarcu D, Isaacson G. Long-term results of endoscopically assisted pediatric cholesteatoma surgery. Otolaryngol Head Neck Surg 2015;154(3):535–9.

12. Haginomori S, Takamaki A, Nonaka R, et al. Residual cholesteatoma: incidence and localization in canal wall down tympanoplasty with soft-wall reconstruction. Arch Otolaryngol Head Neck Surg 2008;134(6):652–7.

13. Barakate M, Bottrill I. Combined approach tympanoplasty for cholesteatoma: impact of middle-ear endoscopy. J Laryngol Otol 2008;122(2):120–4.

14. Thomassin JM, Braccini F. Role of imaging and endoscopy in the follow up and management of cholesteatomas operated by closed technique. Rev Laryngol Otol Rhinol (Bord) 1999;120(2):75–81 [in French].

15. de Zinis LO, Tonni D, Barezzani MG. Single-stage canal wall-down tympanoplasty: long-term results and prognostic factors. Ann Otol Rhinol Laryngol 2010;119(5):304–12.

16. Tomlin J, Chang D, McCutcheon B, et al. Surgical technique and recurrence in cholesteatoma: a meta-analysis. Audiol Neurootol 2013;18(3):135–42.

17. Presutti L, Gioacchini FM, Alicandri-Ciufelli M, et al. Results of endoscopic middle ear surgery for cholesteatoma treatment: a systematic review. Acta Otorhinolaryngol Ital 2014;34(3):153–7.

18. Glasscock ME 3rd, Dickins JR, Wiet R. Cholesteatoma in children. Laryngoscope 1981;91(10):1743–53.

19. Sheehy JL, Brackmann DE, Graham MD. Cholesteatoma surgery: residual and recurrent disease. A review of 1,024 cases. Ann Otol Rhinol Laryngol 1977; 86(4 Pt 1):451–62.

20. Sie KC. Cholesteatoma in children. Pediatr Clin North Am 1996;43(6):1245–52.

21. Rosenberg SI, Silverstein H, Hoffer M, et al. Use of endoscopes for chronic ear surgery in children. Arch Otolaryngol Head Neck Surg 1995;121(8):870–2.

22. Good GM, Isaacson G. Otoendoscopy for improved pediatric cholesteatoma removal. Ann Otol Rhinol Laryngol 1999;108(9):893–6.

23. Marchioni D, Soloperto D, Rubini A, et al. Endoscopic exclusive transcanal approach to the tympanic cavity cholesteatoma in pediatric patients: our experience. Int J Pediatr Otorhinolaryngol 2015;79(3):316–22.

24. Kobayashi T, Gyo K, Komori M, et al. Efficacy and safety of transcanal endoscopic ear surgery for congenital cholesteatomas: a preliminary report. Otol Neurotol 2015;36(10):1644–50.

25. Dornhoffer JL, Friedman AB, Gluth MB. Management of acquired cholesteatoma in the pediatric population. Curr Opin Otolaryngol Head Neck Surg 2013;21(5): 440–5.

26. Chen JM, Schloss MD, Manoukian JJ, et al. Congenital cholesteatoma of the middle ear in children. J Otolaryngol 1989;18(1):44–8.

27. Darrouzet V, Duclos JY, Portmann D, et al. Congenital middle ear cholesteatomas in children: our experience in 34 cases. Otolaryngol Head Neck Surg 2002; 126(1):34–40.

28. Ayache S. Cartilaginous myringoplasty: the endoscopic transcanal procedure. Eur Arch Otorhinolaryngol 2013;270(3):853–60.

29. Furukawa T, Watanabe T, Ito T, et al. Feasibility and advantages of transcanal endoscopic myringoplasty. Otol Neurotol 2014;35(4):e140–5.

30. Tarabichi M, Ayache S, Nogueira JF, et al. Endoscopic management of chronic otitis media and tympanoplasty. Otolaryngol Clin North Am 2013;46(2):155–63.

31. Naik C, Nemade S. Endoscopic stapedotomy: our view point. Eur Arch Otorhinolaryngol 2016;273(1):37–41.

32. Kojima H, Komori M, Chikazawa S, et al. Comparison between endoscopic and microscopic stapes surgery. Laryngoscope 2014;124(1):266–71.

33. Daneshi A, Jahandideh H. Totally endoscopic stapes surgery without packing: novel technique bringing most comfort to the patients. Eur Arch Otorhinolaryngol 2016;273(3):631–4.

34. Marchioni D, Grammatica A, Alicandri-Ciufelli M, et al. Endoscopic cochlear implant procedure. Eur Arch Otorhinolaryngol 2014;271(5):959–66.

35. Marchioni D, Soloperto D, Guarnaccia MC, et al. Endoscopic assisted cochlear implants in ear malformations. Eur Arch Otorhinolaryngol 2015;272(10):2643–52.

36. Migirov L, Shapira Y, Wolf M. The feasibility of endoscopic transcanal approach for insertion of various cochlear electrodes: a pilot study. Eur Arch Otorhinolaryngol 2015;272(7):1637–41.

37. Tarabichi M, Nazhat O, Kassouma J, et al. Endoscopic cochlear implantation: call for caution. Laryngoscope 2015;126(3):689–92.

38. Sun JQ, Sun JW. Endoscope-assisted retrosigmoid keyhole approach for cerebellopontine angle: cadaveric study. Acta Otolaryngol 2013;133(11):1154–7.

39. Pillai P, Sammet S, Ammirati M. Image-guided, endoscopic-assisted drilling and exposure of the whole length of the internal auditory canal and its fundus with preservation of the integrity of the labyrinth using a retrosigmoid approach: a laboratory investigation. Neurosurgery 2009;65(6 Suppl):53–9 [discussion: 59].

40. Kempfle J, Kozin ED, Remenschneider AK, et al. Transcanal retrocochlear approach to the internal auditory canal with cochlear preservation: a pilot cadaveric study. Otolaryngol Head Neck Surg 2016;154(5):920–3.

41. Wackym PA, King WA, Poe DS, et al. Adjunctive use of endoscopy during acoustic neuroma surgery. Laryngoscope 1999;109(8):1193–201.

42. Gerganov VM, Romansky KV, Bussarsky VA, et al. Endoscope-assisted microsurgery of large vestibular schwannomas. Minim Invasive Neurosurg 2005;48(1):39–43.

43. Goksu N, Bayazit Y, Kemaloglu Y. Endoscopy of the posterior fossa and endoscopic dissection of acoustic neuroma. Neurosurg Focus 1999;6(4):e15.

44. Kumon Y, Kohno S, Ohue S, et al. Usefulness of endoscope-assisted microsurgery for removal of vestibular schwannomas. J Neurol Surg B Skull Base 2012;73(1):42–7.

45. Alicandri-Ciufelli M, Marchioni D, Presutti L. The transcanal transpromontorial corridor to treat cochlear schwannomas. Otol Neurotol 2015;36(3):562–3.

46. Presutti L, Alicandri-Ciufelli M, Cigarini E, et al. Cochlear schwannoma removed through the external auditory canal by a transcanal exclusive endoscopic technique. Laryngoscope 2013;123(11):2862–7.

47. Marchioni D, Alicandri-Ciufelli M, Rubini A, et al. Endoscopic transcanal corridors to the lateral skull base: initial experiences. Laryngoscope 2015;125(Suppl 5):S1–13.

48. Carter MS, Lookabaugh S, Lee DJ. Endoscopic-assisted repair of superior canal dehiscence syndrome. Laryngoscope 2014;124(6):1464–8.

49. Shah PV, Kozin ED, Remenschneider AK, et al. Prolonged radiant exposure of the middle ear during transcanal endoscopic ear surgery. Otolaryngol Head Neck Surg 2015;153(1):102–4.

50. Kozin ED, Lehmann A, Carter M, et al. Thermal effects of endoscopy in a human temporal bone model: implications for endoscopic ear surgery. Laryngoscope 2014;124(8):E332–9.

51. MacKeith SA, Frampton S, Pothier DD. Thermal properties of operative endoscopes used in otorhinolaryngology. J Laryngol Otol 2008;122(7):711–4.

52. Nomura K, Oshima H, Yamauchi D, et al. Ototoxic effect of Ultrastop antifog solution applied to the guinea pig middle ear. Otolaryngol Head Neck Surg 2014;151(5):840–4.

53. Thomassin JM, Korchia D, Doris JM. Endoscopic-guided otosurgery in the prevention of residual cholesteatomas. Laryngoscope 1993;103(8):939–43.

54. Youssef TF, Poe DS. Endoscope-assisted second-stage tympanomastoidectomy. Laryngoscope 1997;107(10):1341–4.

55. Haberkamp TJ, Tanyeri H. Surgical techniques to facilitate endoscopic second-look mastoidectomy. Laryngoscope 1999;109(7 Pt 1):1023–7.

56. Badr-el-Dine M. Value of ear endoscopy in cholesteatoma surgery. Otol Neurotol 2002;23(5):631–5.

57. El-Meselaty K, Badr-El-Dine M, Mandour M, et al. Endoscope affects decision making in cholesteatoma surgery. Otolaryngol Head Neck Surg 2003;129(5):490–6.

58. Ayache S, Tramier B, Strunski V. Otoendoscopy in cholesteatoma surgery of the middle ear: what benefits can be expected? Otol Neurotol 2008;29(8):1085–90.

59. Presutti L, Marchioni D, Mattioli F, et al. Endoscopic management of acquired cholesteatoma: our experience. J Otolaryngol Head Neck Surg 2008;37(4):481–7.

60. Yung MM. The use of rigid endoscopes in cholesteatoma surgery. J Laryngol Otol 1994;108(4):307–9.

61. Bottrill ID, Poe DS. Endoscope-assisted ear surgery. Am J Otol 1995;16(2):158–63.

62. Yung MW. The use of middle ear endoscopy: has residual cholesteatoma been eliminated? J Laryngol Otol 2001;115(12):958–61.

63. Tarabichi M. Endoscopic management of limited attic cholesteatoma. Laryngoscope 2004;114(7):1157–62.

64. Marchioni D, Mattioli F, Alicandri-Ciufelli M, et al. Endoscopic approach to tensor fold in patients with attic cholesteatoma. Acta Otolaryngol 2009;129(9):946–54.

65. Migirov L, Shapira Y, Horowitz Z, et al. Exclusive endoscopic ear surgery for acquired cholesteatoma: preliminary results. Otol Neurotol 2011;32(3):433–6.

66. Marchioni D, Alicandri-Ciufelli M, Molteni G, et al. Ossicular chain preservation after exclusive endoscopic transcanal tympanoplasty: preliminary experience. Otol Neurotol 2011;32(4):626–31.

67. Marchioni D, Villari D, Mattioli F, et al. Endoscopic management of attic cholesteatoma: a single-institution experience. Otolaryngol Clin North Am 2013;46(2):201–9.

68. Hanna BM, Kivekas I, Wu YH, et al. Minimally invasive functional approach for cholesteatoma surgery. Laryngoscope 2014;124(10):2386–92.

69. el-Guindy A. Endoscopic transcanal myringoplasty. J Laryngol Otol 1992;106(6):493–5.

70. Usami S, Iijima N, Fujita S, et al. Endoscopic-assisted myringoplasty. ORL J Otorhinolaryngol Relat Spec 2001;63(5):287–90.

71. Jang CH, Kim YH, Cho YB, et al. Endoscopy-aided laser therapy for intractable granular myringitis. J Laryngol Otol 2006;120(7):553–5.

72. Kakehata S, Futai K, Sasaki A, et al. Endoscopic transtympanic tympanoplasty in the treatment of conductive hearing loss: early results. Otol Neurotol 2006;27(1):14–9.

73. Yadav SP, Aggarwal N, Julaha M, et al. Endoscope-assisted myringoplasty. Singapore Med J 2009;50(5):510–2.

74. Marchioni D, Alicandri-Ciufelli M, Molteni G, et al. Endoscopic tympanoplasty in patients with attic retraction pockets. Laryngoscope 2010;120(9):1847–55.
75. Konstantinidis I, Malliari H, Tsakiropoulou E, et al. Fat myringoplasty outcome analysis with otoendoscopy: who is the suitable patient? Otol Neurotol 2013; 34(1):95–9.
76. Marchioni D, Alicandri-Ciufelli M, Gioacchini FM, et al. Transcanal endoscopic treatment of benign middle ear neoplasms. Eur Arch Otorhinolaryngol 2013; 270(12):2997–3004.

Size as a Risk Factor for Growth in Conservatively Managed Vestibular Schwannomas

The Birmingham Experience

Charles R.J. Daultrey, MRCS[a],*, James W. Rainsbury, FRCS[a,b], Richard M. Irving, FRCS[a]

KEYWORDS

• Vestibular schwannoma • Tumor • Growth • Size

INTRODUCTION

Vestibular schwannoma (VS) is a benign primary intracranial tumor of the myelin-forming cells of the vestibulocochlear nerve, representing about 6% of all intracranial tumors.[1] The neuromas usually manifest with unilateral hearing impairment, which may go unnoticed by the patient or clinician. Early diagnosis offers patients a range of management options and may significantly reduce morbidity.[1]

The incidence of acoustic neuromas is around 13 cases/million/y, with peaks in the fifth and sixth decades of life, affecting both sexes equally.[2,3] Estimates of prevalence have so far been calculated only from large, unselected autopsy or radiology studies, with a suggested figure of 0.8%.[4]

Advances in MRI have allowed the discovery of these tumors earlier in the disease process and with more sensitivity. With reducing cost and increasing MRI availability, screening has become standard practice in patients with unilateral audiovestibular symptoms. Current published literature corroborates this increase in the diagnosis of small tumors and a decrease in the number of diagnosed large and medium-sized neuromas.[5–8]

The management strategy for VS is multifactorial, influenced by size, patient age, general health, extent of hearing loss, and the patient's own preference. With the shift to smaller tumors at diagnosis, a more conservative approach to management has been seen, allowing the observation of tumor natural history with serial scanning. Active treatment with stereotactic radiotherapy (SRT) or surgical resection may be

Conflicts of Interest and Source of Funding: None to declare.
[a] University Hospital Birmingham, Birmingham, UK; [b] Derriford Hospital, Plymouth, UK
* Corresponding author. 55, Station Road, Birmingham, West Midlands B17 9LP, UK.
E-mail address: c.daultrey@doctors.org.uk

Otolaryngol Clin N Am 49 (2016) 1291–1295
http://dx.doi.org/10.1016/j.otc.2016.08.002

oto.theclinics.com

delayed using a watch-and-wait policy, although this does give rise to a greater patient load and strain on resources, whereas earlier diagnosis adds to patient stress and concerns regarding growth and potential intervention.[9]

Understanding growth in conservatively managed tumors would allow better understanding of which tumors are more likely to grow, and the development of tailored imaging protocols depending on tumor characteristics and likelihood of progression. This understanding would allow optimal resource use; it would improve clinicians' ability to counsel patients as to their tumor growth prognosis; and the treatment pathway could be streamlined so that interventions, such as SRT, could be instigated earlier for tumors known to grow more aggressively.

This case series explores tumors observed in conservatively managed patients seen in a large tertiary center VS clinic service at Queen Elizabeth Hospital, Birmingham (QEHB). The authors observed whether tumor size at presentation was associated with subsequent growth rate.

METHOD

A retrospective case note review was performed using a large database containing more than 900 patients with VS managed at QEHB between 1997 and 2012. Patients from this database with tumors up to 2 cm at the cerebellopontine angle (CPA) were included because most of this group was initially managed conservatively at our unit. For the purpose of analysis, tumors were arbitrarily divided into 3 groups: those with predominant intracanalicular (IC) component, and extracanalicular tumors measuring 1 to 10 mm or 11 to 20 mm at the CPA.

Serial scans were performed as per the local protocol described by Martin and colleagues[6]: after initial diagnostic MRI, scans are repeated at 6 months after diagnosis, then at annual intervals for 2 years. A further scan is performed 2 years later, then every 5 years for life. Scans were reviewed by a single individual, to avoid interoperator variability, with measurements taken across the face of the petrous temporal bones.

Tumors that had shown more than 1-mm increase in diameter over any number of serial images were deemed to be growing. The main outcome measures of interest were the proportion (%) of tumors that had grown in each study group, and the mean growth rate of this subgroup of growing tumors (millimeters per year; measured over the duration of follow-up for a tumor).

Statistical analysis was performed using Microsoft Excel 2010. A χ^2-test was performed to compare the proportion of growing tumors between groups, and an unpaired, 1-tailed t-test to compare mean annual growth rates for the growing tumor subsets.

RESULTS

Five-hundred and fifty-five patients were included in the study, with 287 men and 268 women. There were 265 intracanalicular tumors, 154 tumors measuring from 1 to 10 mm and 136 tumors from 11 to 20 mm at the CPA. Demographics, along with tumor sizes and growth rates observed, are shown in **Table 1**. Of the growing tumors, those in the 11-mm to 20-mm group grew the fastest, followed by the 1-mm to 10-mm group, and then the IC tumors.

IC tumors were less likely to grow than either group of EC tumors ($P<.01$; **Table 2**). Growing tumors in the 11-mm to 20-mm group grew faster than the IC subset ($P = .04$), but not compared with the 1-mm to 10-mm subset ($P = .08$); there was no difference in growth rate between IC and 1-mm to 10-mm subsets ($P = .30$) (Table 3).

Table 1
Tumor demographics and characteristics

	Male	Female	Mean CPA Diameter (mm)	Number Grown	% Grown	Mean Growth Rate (mm/y)
IC	141	124	NA	15	5.7	3.3
1–10	78	76	7	28	18.2	3.8
11–20	68	68	15	23	16.9	5.3
Total	287	268	—	66	11.9	4.2

Abbreviation: NA, not applicable.

DISCUSSION

This series sought to observe whether tumor size at presentation related to growth. EC tumors were significantly more likely to grow than IC tumors, and increased size at presentation in EC tumors is associated with growth rates.

With publication of Stangerup and colleagues'[5] article in 2006 on the natural history of VS, which found that only a small number of tumors grew within the first 5 years, many centers have developed a more conservative approach to managing small tumors and observation protocols for such VS were established.

This shift toward conservative management has increased with earlier detection of smaller VSs, whereas improvements in MRI techniques have further increased diagnostic sensitivity.[10,11] Patel and colleagues'[12] recent 2014 review confirmed this, with their national cancer center registry Surveillance Epidemiology and End Results (SEER) database, revealing similar results to the Stangerup and colleagues[5] study and others examining tumor growth. Patel and colleagues[12] observed that, in the United States, tumor size at diagnosis decreased significantly (1966–1998, 23.8% ≤1.5 cm; 1999–2008, 45.3% ≤1.5 cm).

In Stangerup and colleagues[5] study (552 patients), 17% of the IC tumors grew, whereas significantly ($P<.001$) more of the EC tumors displayed growth during the study period (28.9%). In our 555-patient series only 5.7% of IC tumors grew versus 17.6% of EC tumors, but, in keeping with Stangerup and colleagues'[5] results, the EC tumors in our series were more likely to grow than IC tumors.

Hughes and colleagues[13] conducted a retrospective observational study assessing the consequences of conservative management of VS with data collected from tertiary neuro-otological referral units in the United Kingdom. The study included 59 patients who were managed conservatively and, similar to our data, found that tumors extending into the CPA at diagnosis grow significantly faster than those confined to the internal auditory meatus, referred to as IC tumors in our series.

No other reliable predictors of tumor growth were identified through Hughes and colleagues'[13] study; they commented that no association with growth rate was found

Table 2
Tumor percentage growth as a comparison

χ^2 Comparing Tumor % Grown	
IC vs 1–10	<0.01
IC vs 11–20	<0.01
1–10 vs 11–20	0.77

Table 3
Tumor growth rates as a comparison (1 tailed, unequal variance)

t-Test Comparing Mean Growth Rates	
IC vs 1–10	0.30
IC vs 11–20	0.04
1–10 vs 11–20	0.08

when assessing age, sex, laterality of tumor, and selected clinical findings (VII and VIII nerve function) at the time of diagnosis. Their literature review gave inconsistent results but did not identify useful predictors of growth. Similarly, Bedersen and colleagues,[14] Flint and colleagues,[15] Rosenberg,[16] and Walsh and colleagues[17] found no correlation between growth and initial symptoms, initial size, duration of symptoms, laterality, gender, and age.

Published literature to date, including systematic review and meta-analysis, has predominantly found slow VS tumor growth in conservatively managed patients, ranging from 0.66 to 1.9 mm/y.[13,18–21] These series included all study tumors when considering growth rates, including those deemed to be not growing, and showed comparable results with our observed growths; when our nongrowing tumors are included in the calculation, IC tumors grew at a rate of 0.2 mm/y, whereas EC tumors categorized as 1–10 mm and 11–20 mm grew 0.7 and 0.9 mm/y, respectively.

Martin and colleagues'[6] findings of 4 mm/y annual growth (range, 0.5–17 mm/y) in growing tumors compares with our study finding of 4.2 mm/y when nongrowing tumors are removed from the series.

This 555-strong case series agrees with current literature; EC tumors of any size at presentation are more likely to grow than IC tumors, and growth rates and size changes are similar to those published currently.

SUMMARY

This series shows that larger EC tumors grow faster than IC tumors and that EC tumors overall at presentation are more likely to grow than IC tumors.

With this observed disparity in growth pattern, it may be that screening programs such as that of Martin and colleagues[6] can be modified to consider the slower growing processes observed in IC tumors, thus reducing scan regularity and strain on department resources and funds.

With improved tumor growth pattern understanding, patient counseling at diagnosis can be improved; for example, by considering more conservative screening in IC tumors, and possibly earlier intervention in those larger EC tumors with more aggressive growth potential.

REFERENCES

1. British Association of Otorhinolaryngologists, Head and Neck Surgeons. Clinical effectiveness guidelines for acoustic neuroma. British Association of Otorhinolaryngologists, Head and Neck Surgeons; 2002. Available at: www.entuk.org/members/publications/ceg_acousticneuroma.pdf.
2. Moffat DA, Hardy DO, Baguley DM. Strategy and benefits of acoustic neuroma searching. J Laryngol Otol 1989;103:51–9.
3. Davis AC. Some aspects of the epidemiology of acoustic neuromas. Proc. Acoustic Neuroma Meeting. Nottingham, 1995.

4. Leonard JR, Talbot ML. Asymptomatic acoustic neurilemmoma. Arch Otolaryngol 1970;91:117–24.
5. Stangerup SE, Caye-Thomasen P, Tos M, et al. The natural history of vestibular schwannoma. Otol Neurotol 2006;27:547–52.
6. Martin TP, Senthil L, Chavda SV, et al. A protocol for the conservative management of vestibular schwannomas. Otol Neurotol 2009;30(3):381–5.
7. Hajioff D, Raut VV, Walsh RM, et al. Conservative management of vestibular schwannomas: third review of a 10-year prospective study. Clin Otolaryngol 2008;33:255–9.
8. Battaglia A, Mastrodimos B, Cueva R. Comparison of growth patterns of acoustic neuromas with and without radiosurgery. Otol Neurotol 2006;27:705–12.
9. Vogel JJ, Godefroy WP, van der Mey AG, et al. Illness perceptions, coping, and quality of life in vestibular schwannoma patients at diagnosis. Otol Neurotol 2008; 29(6):839–45.
10. Stangerup SE, Tos M, Thomsen J, et al. True incidence of vestibular schwannoma? Neurosurgery 2010;67:1335–40 [discussion: 1340].
11. Evans DG, Moran A, King A, et al. Incidence of vestibular schwannoma and neurofibromatosis 2 in the North West of England over a 10-year period: higher incidence than previously thought. Otol Neurotol 2005;26:93–7.
12. Patel J, Vasan R, Van Loveren H, et al. The changing face of acoustic neuroma management in the USA: analysis of the 1998 and 2008 patient surveys from the acoustic neuroma association. Br J Neurosurg 2014;28(1):20–4.
13. Hughes M, Skilbeck C, Saeed S, et al. Expectant management of vestibular schwannoma: a retrospective multivariate analysis of tumour growth and outcome. Skull Base 2011;21(5):295–302.
14. Bederson JB, von Ammon K, Wichmann W, et al. Conservative treatment of patients with acoustic tumors. Neurosurgery 1991;28(5):646–50 [discussion: 650–1].
15. Flint D, Fagan P, Panarese A. Conservative management of sporadic unilateral acoustic neuromas. J Laryngol Otol 2005;119(6):424–8.
16. Rosenberg SI. Natural history of acoustic neuromas. Laryngoscope 2000;110(4): 497–508.
17. Walsh RM, Bath AP, Bance ML, et al. Consequences to hearing during the conservative management of vestibular schwannomas. Laryngoscope 2000;110(2 Pt 1):250–5.
18. Yamakami I, Uchino Y, Kobayashi E, et al. Conservative management, gamma-knife radiosurgery, and micro- surgery for acoustic neurinomas: a systematic review of outcome and risk of three therapeutic options. Neurol Res 2003;25(7): 682–90.
19. Yoshimoto Y. Systematic review of the natural history of vestibular schwannoma. J Neurosurg 2005;103(1):59–63.
20. Smouha EE, Yoo M, Mohr K, et al. Conservative management of acoustic neuroma: a meta-analysis and proposed treatment algorithm. Laryngoscope 2005; 115(3):450–4.
21. Selesnick SH, Johnson G. Radiologic surveillance of acoustic neuromas. Am J Otol 1998;19(6):846–9.

Index

Note: Page numbers of article titles are in **boldface** type.

Otolaryngol Clin N Am 49 (2016) 1297–1301
http://dx.doi.org/10.1016/S0030-6665(16)30136-0
0030-6665/16/$ – see front matter

Moving?

Make sure your subscription moves with you!

To notify us of your new address, find your **Clinics Account Number** (located on your mailing label above your name), and contact customer service at:

Email: journalscustomerservice-usa@elsevier.com

800-654-2452 (subscribers in the U.S. & Canada)
314-447-8871 (subscribers outside of the U.S. & Canada)

Fax number: 314-447-8029

Elsevier Health Sciences Division
Subscription Customer Service
3251 Riverport Lane
Maryland Heights, MO 63043

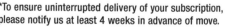

*To ensure uninterrupted delivery of your subscription, please notify us at least 4 weeks in advance of move.

Printed and bound by CPI Group (UK) Ltd, Croydon, CR0 4YY

03/10/2024

01040394-0002